POCKET PSYCHIATRY

SECOND EDITION

Commissioning Editor: Miranda Bromage
Project Development Manager: Tim Kimber
Project Manager: Katharine Eyston
Design Manager: Andy Chapman
Designer: Keith Kail

POCKET PSYCHIATRY

SECOND EDITION

Kamaldeep Bhui MD, MSc, MRCPsych, DipClinPsych

Senior Lecturer in Social and Epidemiological Psychiatry, Department of Psychiatry, Barts and London Medical School, Queen Mary University of London, London

Scott Weich MD, MSc, MRCPsych

Senior Lecturer in Psychiatry, Department of Psychiatry and Behavioural Sciences, Royal Free and University College Medical School; Honorary Consultant Psychiatrist, Camden and Islington Mental Health NHS Trust, London

Keith Lloyd MD, MSc, MRCPsych

Senior Lecturer, Department of Mental Health, University of Exeter and Consultant Psychiatrist, Devon Partnership NHS Trust, Exeter

Foreword by

Graham Thornicroft

Professor of Community Psychiatry, Institute of Psychiatry, London

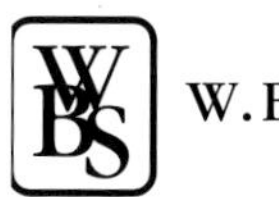

W.B. SAUNDERS

London Edinburgh New York Philadelphia St Louis Sydney Toronto 2002

WB SAUNDERS
An imprint of Harcourt Publishers Limited

First published 2002

ISBN 0 7020 2631 X

British Library Cataloguing in Publication Data
A catalogue record for this book is available from the British Library

Library of Congress Cataloging in Publication Data
A catalog record for this book is available from the Library of Congress

Drug Nomenclature
Directive 92/27/EEC requires use of the Recommended International Non-proprietary Name (rINN) for medicinal substances. In most cases the British Approved Name (BAN) and rINN are identical but where they differ the rINN has been used.

Drug Dosages
Medical knowledge is constantly changing. As new information becomes available, changes in treatment, procedures, equipment and the use of drugs become necessary. The editors/authors/contributors and the publishers have taken care to ensure that the information given in this text is accurate and up to date. However, readers are strongly advised to confirm that the information, especially with regard to drug usage, complies with the latest legislation and standards of practice.

The Publisher's policy is to use **paper manufactured from sustainable forests**

Printed in China by RDC Group Limited

Contents

Contributors

Anne Aubin
Consultant Child and Adolescent Psychiatrist, Plymouth Hospitals Trust, Plymouth, UK

Kamaldeep Bhui
Senior Lecturer in Social and Epidemiological Psychiatry, Department of Psychiatry, Barts and London Medical School, Queen Mary University of London, London, UK

Navina Evans
Consultant Child and Adolescent Psychiatrist, East London and City Mental Health Trust, London, UK

Tim Hardie
Consultant Forensic Psychiatrist, East Midlands Centre for Forensic Mental Health, Leicester, UK

Anne Lingford-Hughes
Senior Lecturer in Biological Psychiatry and Addiction, Division of Psychiatry, University of Bristol, Bristol, UK

Keith Lloyd
Senior Lecturer, Department of Mental Health, University of Exeter and Consultant Psychiatrist, Devon Partnership NHS Trust, Exeter, UK

Carol Paton
Principal Pharmacist, Bexley Hospital, Bexley, Kent, UK

Ioana Popescu
Specialist Registrar in Old Age Psychiatry, Department of Mental Health Care for Older People, East London and the City Mental Health NHS Trust, Homerton Hospital, London, UK

Alison Puffet
Consultant Psychiatrist, London, UK

Kim Sutherby
Consultant Psychiatrist, South London and Maudsley Trust, London, UK

Scott Weich
Senior Lecturer in Psychiatry, Department of Psychiatry and Behavioural Sciences, Royal Free and University College Medical School; Honorary Consultant Psychiatrist, Camden and Islington Mental Health NHS Trust, London, UK

Foreword

Fairly or not, psychiatrists often feel much maligned. One of my favourite jokes about the profession reflects a view of the psychiatrist as something less than a serious practitioner and describes a man who goes to see a psychiatrist. 'Doc, I keep having these alternating recurring dreams. First I'm a teepee; then I'm a wigwam; then I'm a teepee; then I'm a wigwam. It's driving me crazy. What's wrong with me?' The doctor replies: 'It's very simple. You're two tents!'

In fact, the degree of clinical and scientific rigour required of British trainee psychiatrists to qualify to be a consultant is now on a par with any other medical discipline; many people do not realise that it takes at least seven years to qualify as a specialist after the completion of undergraduate medical student training. GPs, social workers, nurses and support workers also seek excellence in mental health care. Mental health professionals need to find a fusion between dealing with patients in a compassionate, considered and respectful way, and applying up-to-date technical knowledge about the nature of the conditions they recognize and using the best available treatments to relieve distress and suffering.

In the course of higher professional training, but also in practice, clinicians need to refer to a succinct source of information that is directly relevant to the immediate clinical question they need to answer. All clinicians, regardless of seniority and discipline, are developing evidence-based practice skills for the care of the mentally ill.

Pocket Psychiatry exactly fulfils this role. In the tradition of the 'vade mecum' (a handbook carried constantly for use), this is an elegant and select summary of what the modern clinician needs to know, whatever the situation. As relevant to an emergency home visit or Mental Health Act assessment in a police station as it is to a planned appointment for a session of psychotherapy, this book is practical, polished and punchy. All three editors are experienced clinicians as well as accomplished academics, and it is this blend of expertise and experience that lends the text its twin hallmarks: it is both authoritative and genuinely useful. This second edition brings the text up to date and reflects the changing nature of evidence and policy in the field of mental health, while maintaining the clarity and compression that marked the successful first edition. It is a jewel of a book, which reflects the exclamation of Shakespeare in *Hamlet*:

> A cut-purse of the empire and the rule,
> That from a shelf the precious diadem stole,
> And put it in his pocket!

Graham Thornicroft
Professor of Community Psychiatry, Sir David Goldberg Centre for Health Services Research, Institute of Psychiatry, London
25 September 2002

Preface

Pocket Psychiatry collates clinically relevant information for practitioners working with the mentally ill. This is the second edition. Its production was stimulated again by extensive discussion with students and colleagues. The previous edition has now been strengthened by a number of contributors on specialist areas of practice. There is a forensic psychiatry section, a much fuller child and adolescent psychiatry section, and a section on psychiatry in later life, as well as revised sections on substance misuse, alcohol, neuroimaging and psychiatry, drug treatments, obstetrics and gynaecology, and eating disorders. We have had positive feedback from general practitioners, students and psychiatric trainees. The text is also valuable to members of multidisciplinary mental health teams and primary care teams as it summarizes clinically relevant information for psychiatric practice. We have made this second edition more accessible to a wider audience so that it is enjoyable to use on an everyday basis. Learning should be enjoyable as well as informative. Enjoy *Pocket Psychiatry*.

Kam Bhui
Scott Weich
Keith Lloyd

Acknowledgements

To family, friends, students, colleagues and service users who stimulated and supported our work. *Pocket Psychiatry* would not exist without them.

SECTION I

Assessment

THE PSYCHIATRIC ASSESSMENT

An overview of the necessary information from the history and mental state examination is presented below. This aims to serve as an *aide mémoire* for the commonest types of problem areas but is not comprehensive. A more detailed overview can be obtained from the major textbooks on psychiatry and psychopathology[1–3] and the descriptive psychopathology section (p. 254).

THE PSYCHIATRIC HISTORY

BASIC INFORMATION

Name, age, sex, first language, ethnicity, religion, address, telephone number, occupation.

Names and telephone numbers of:

- Any health-care professional involved in care: GP, psychiatrists, psychologists
- Any social services professionals involved in care: social worker, probation officer
- Any voluntary organizations involved in care: housing, education, leisure
- Family/friends who can provide immediate support and corroborative information.

PRESENTING PROBLEMS

- According to patient
- According to family
- According to neighbours, friends, police, landlords, etc.

For each problem/symptom elicit:

- Duration, onset, maximal/minimal intensity, periodicity, triggers
- Aggravating factors and alleviating factors: classify as biological, social, psychological
- Detailed account of most recent symptoms/problems which led to seeking help
- Any evidence of depression, major psychoses, suicidality?
- What interventions and coping strategies has the patient already used?
- What interventions and coping strategies were unsuccessful and why?

SOCIAL CIRCUMSTANCES

Housing

Cost, quality, crowding, contented?

Employment

Duration, stability, recent functioning.

Financial

Income and debts.

Relationship

Married? Long-term partner? Any difficulties recently?

Life events

Bereavements, loss of work, stressors, relationship problems, any recent significant changes of circumstance.

FAMILY HISTORY

Family psychiatric diagnoses, contact with hospitals (medical and psychiatric), treatments used, current level of contact with index patient, current state of psychiatric illness, occupations, proximity. Identify any unexplained deaths, sudden death associated with alcohol, potential suicides and any evidence that relatives had a mental illness.

Relationship with siblings and parents, trusting relationships, any trusts broken? Closeness, amount of contact, effective social support provided? Separations – how were they managed?

Other children: ages, schooling, development, academic progress, illness – specific nervous problems, any evidence of conduct disorder, severe unhappiness – contact with social services, hospitals, GP.

PERSONAL HISTORY

Childhood

Information from memory, family or reports. Early indicators of personality traits. Life events – unhappiness. Include physical illness, neurotic traits such as fears/phobia. Academic and social progress, special needs school? Truancy, school phobia, bullying, victimization for other reasons (obesity, race, size, etc.). Try to obtain old school reports, psychological assessments and any other data. Timing of school changes, reasons for, adjustments to changes, friendships.

- Place and date of birth
- Family size and birth order
- Early childhood
  - Childhood illness
  - Developmental delays
  - Schooling
  - Changing school

Adolescence

Hobbies, ambitions, personality, life events, academic record, unhappiness, relationships, sexual experience, negotiating puberty and sexual development, relationship with peers, teachers, relatives and parents.

Adulthood

First job, length of occupations subsequently, reasons for change of job, problems with authority, colleagues, family and friends. Life events. Relationship successes and failures (include reasons for). List all major relationships, duration, specific problems, how they ended – any pattern? Marriages, children, sexual functioning during and between relationships, sexual victimization, sexual offences (if relevant) and fantasy life. Hobbies, sports, social, special skills, any achievements.

- Employment
- Relationship
- Leisure

Past psychiatric and medical history

List past hospital admissions, operations, illness, treatments, starting with most recent. Obtain records if possible from previous admission and treatment episodes. If information lacking contact previous Responsible Medical Officers (RMOs: the consultant). Results from previous investigations can save much time and prevent unnecessary repeat investigations.

Personality

Elicit patient's self-report of strengths and weaknesses, how they start and end relationships. Ask about any good friends, did they have pets in childhood, did they have any meaningful relationships, how do they deal with frustration, anger, aggression, jealousy, episodes of sadness, low self-esteem? How does the patient perceive that others treat them? Criminality, special skills and abilities. Obtain informant history: GP, friend, partner, family member. Identify any maladaptive recurrent patterns of behaviour, when they arose and the negative consequences. Does the patient identify any aspects of their behaviour as problematic either for their social or occupational functioning? Is there any evidence that the patient can change their behaviour on the basis of previous experience? There are some simple structured instruments (often self-report) that will help with the assessment of personality (for example Ryle's *Psychotherapy File*).[4]

Medication

List all current medications, their indications, any adverse effects that the patient experienced, previous medications and reasons for stopping. Record any drugs to which patient has had adverse or allergic responses. Note how reliably the patient can recall this information and how frequently and to what extent the patient varies their medication regimen.

Substances of abuse

Obtain detailed information about the specific drugs used, why they need the drug. The amount, the duration of effect, the adverse effects experienced, associated criminal activities, associated financial difficulties, the cost, escalation in use, contact with hospitals, administration routes, clean needle use. HIV/hepatitis B/C status. Previous treatment episodes in or out of hospital, detoxification strategies used. Prescribed maintenance regimens? Specific names and addresses of doctors, therapists and clinics must be corroborated. Every aspect of the history needs to be corroborated – drug craving and associated financial difficulties encourage addicts to obtain drugs by any means possible.

Alcohol use

When they started drinking alcohol, how much, what they drink, when they take a drink. At what time of day they take a first drink. Any evidence of tolerance (needing more and more alcohol) and withdrawal symptoms? Are there social, forensic and physical health-care sequelae? Periods of abstinence and attempts at controlling drinking. Previous treatments, the intensity of treatments and the effectiveness of them. Which might work again if applied?

Forensic history

Identify any previous criminal convictions, the exact nature of the offence (e.g. weapons, injuries to self or others), any prison sentences served, duration of sentences, any psychiatric assessments at the time, ever diverted from court or prison to hospital under Mental Health Act order; were admissions to regional secure units or district hospitals? Try to identify specifically courts, forensic psychiatrists and prisons where the patient was assessed.

MENTAL STATE EXAMINATION

APPEARANCE

Clothes (clean, old, inappropriate for weather, sexually revealing), smoking, gait, level of consciousness, coordination over limbs, mannerism, stereotypies, agitation, tremor and parkinsonian symptoms (bradykinesia, rigidity – cogwheeling), torticollis, dystonias, tardive dyskinesia, facial expression (frowning, sad, blunted, smiling, incongruous with emotions). Physical disabilities, scars, visible cuts on arms, needle marks visible, tattoos. Smell of alcohol.

BEHAVIOUR

Overactivity, underactivity, stuporose, attacking others, able to hold conversation, frightened, staring into corners of the room, preoccupied by internal experience, perplexed, long pauses in answering questions, distractible, wringing hands, pacing around the room, sitting and then standing, invading personal space, sexually inappropriate, threatening, unpredictable. Might they be intoxicated with alcohol or drugs?

MOOD

Expansive, elated, grandiose, overfamiliar, laughing infectiously, irritable, angry, anxious; rapid changes of mood and unable to engage in any conversation. Restricted range of emotional expression? Assess ability to feel remorse, presence of guilt. Do any preoccupations suggest depression (e.g. poverty, worthlessness, helplessness, morbid fears about body function, suicidal ideas, hopelessness)?

SPEECH AND THOUGHTS

Dysarthria or dysphasia – fluent or non-fluent (see reference 3 for a detailed discussion of dysphasias) Comment on form, flow and content. **Form**: thought disordered, 'knight's move' thinking, flight of ideas, circumstantiality. **Flow**: pressure of speech, hesitant, interrupted by distraction, word-finding difficulties, logoclonia, echolalia. **Content**: neologisms, paraphasia, bizarre beliefs (see below), illogicality.

Thought interference from outside agencies (thought insertion), thought blocking (snapping off; thought withdrawal), broadcast, fusion, muddling, concrete thinking, overinclusive thinking.

PERCEPTIONS

Hallucinations (true and pseudo): visual, auditory, somatic, gustatory, olfactory. Hypnagogic, hypnopompic, functional, reflex, extracampine. Depersonalization, derealization, illusions, imagery.

BELIEFS

Delusions: systematized, simple, monosymptomatic, or overvalued idea. Culturally sanctioned and religious beliefs can sometimes be misunderstood as indications of illness. If any unusual beliefs are elicited, evaluate how their reality may be tested. How does the patient respond to the suggestion that you wish to check out the details and evidence? How did these beliefs arise: what persuaded the patient that what they believe is true? How does the patient appraise evidence that is inconsistent with the content of the beliefs?

ANXIETY SYMPTOMS

Obsessional thinking, compulsive behaviour, panic attacks, phobic avoidance of places, people, animals, situations. Overaware of bodily functions. Observe sweating, tremor, fearful affect.

PERSONAL EXPLANATION AND INSIGHT

Ask the following questions:

- Does the patient have any unusual experiences?
- Could these be signs of illness?
- Has the patient's behaviour altered recently?
- Have any of their friends, family, church, etc. noticed this change?
- Has this change brought them into any conflict with people?
- Is the change desirable?
- Is it indicative of illness?
- Do any of the changes in thinking and behaviour constitute a recognized disorder that falls within the domains of psychological functioning?
- Do they need treatment for this illness?
- Will they accept treatment (physical, i.e. drugs; psychotherapeutic; social circumstances need to change)?

Finally, when prescribed treatments or interventions are arranged the clinician needs to make a judgement about how well the patient's actual adherence is reflected by their verbal reports about compliance.

COGNITIVE ASSESSMENT*

- **Orientation**: time, place, personal. Age, date of birth, floor, building, people around (who are they?)
- **Attention and concentration**: registration of information: ask patient to repeat a number; increase the number of digits until they can no longer do this. Most people can manage seven items. Repeat with a seven-item number or name and address
- **Memory**: 5 minutes following registration, test memory of seven-item name and address (do not warn the patient that you are testing memory otherwise they will rehearse)
  – *Remote memory*: account of their life and major public events during their lifetime and news within the preceding weeks
  – *Visual memory* can be tested by asking patient to draw/copy certain shapes, hiding them and asking patient to reproduce them after 5 minutes
- **Language**: naming objects, fingers – nominal aphasia is an early sign of dementia. Give a written (needs to be read by subject) and verbal two- and three-stage commands. This tests comprehension (receptive dysphasia?) but also whether sequences of activity can be carried out. Agraphia

* For patients with neuropsychiatric disorders a much more thorough assessment is required (see reference 5).

is an inability to write, alexia is inability to read.[6] From the subject's speech and conversation during the interview one can make a judgement about the presence of dysphasia or dysarthria

- **Intelligence**: simple arithmetic or serial sevens; some idea of IQ can be obtained from historical reports (school or psychology)
- **Spatial awareness**: draw a clock face, place hands on it. Copying a star, cube, cat or abstract design. Can patient find their way around the ward, building, local area?

TESTING CENTRAL NERVOUS SYSTEM FUNCTIONS

- **Frontal lobe tasks**: sequences of behaviour, e.g. place your fist on the table, now the edge of the hand and now the flat of the hand; repeat this and continue doing so (Luria's test). Ask for the same with the other hand. As in the mini-mental state:[7] take this piece of paper, fold it in half and place it on the floor. Ask for test to be done with both hands. Interpretation of proverbs also used. Verbal fluency also used: say as many words beginning with the letter T or name as many four-legged animals as possible. Apathy, lability of mood, poor motivation and loss of social graces, disinhibition, irritability, perseverative utilization behaviour, urinary incontinence are also indicative of frontal pathology. Inferior frontal gyrus (dominant lobe) lesion affects Broca's area, causing non-fluent dysphasia
- **Temporal lobe tasks**: non-dominant lesion affects visual memory, e.g. prosopagnosia. Dominant lesion affects verbal memory, and sensory deficits such as alexia, agraphia and aphasia arise. Receptive aphasia usually presents as word salad and indicates Wernicke's area lesion (dominant lobe). Musical agnosia. Bilateral lesions cause amnestic syndromes
- **Parietal lobe tasks**: aphasia, astereognosis, two-point discrimination (normally 2 mm at fingertips). Gerstmann's syndrome when a dominant lobe lesion: dyscalculia, left/right disorientation, finger agnosia. Loss of spatial awareness (drawing a star, etc.), dressing apraxia, hemineglect, altered body image (these usually with a non-dominant-lobe lesion)
- **Occipital lobe tasks**: cortical blindness, colour agnosia. Anton's syndrome (vertebrobasilar occlusion) causes loss of vision but a denial of the deficit

PHYSICAL STATUS

A brief selective physical examination should always be carried out if any of the history or mental state or patient's self-reported symptoms indicate the possibility of organic illness. The following summary is a quick overview of potential psychiatric presentation with underlying organic illness.

PHYSICAL EXAMINATION

- **Head and neck**: blood stains, scalp lacerations, neck movements, evidence of head injury, facial symmetry, neck lumps, facial colour (pallor or flushing), telangiectasia (alcohol-related?), jaundice, complexion, rash, lid lag, exophthalmos, squint, gaze palsies, visual fields. Cuts, bruises, orofacial movement disorders
- **Eyes**: pupils: equal size, dilated (anxiety and opiate withdrawal, anticholinergics) or pinpoint (opiate intoxication). Examine fundi if any indication of poor sight, metabolic or arterial disorder or neuropsychiatric presentation. Ophthalmoplegia (Wernicke's encephalopathy)
- **Hands**: nicotine stains, nail length and cleanliness, pitting (psoriasis), evidence of cardiovascular, respiratory or metabolic disorders (clubbing, small infarcts – one of the signs of subacute bacterial endocarditis, which may arise in injecting opiate addicts), koilonychia, rheumatoid nodules and osteoarthritis (Heberden's nodes; indicate possibility of chronic pain). Tremor. Dupuytren's contracture (alcohol, phenytoin toxicity, palmar erythema – alcohol-related)
- **Pulse rate**: *Increased*: anxiety, thyrotoxicosis. *Slow*: hypothyroid states, beta-blockers
- **Respiratory rate**: anxiety, asthma, heart failure, traumatic chest injury
- **Blood pressure**: low because of antiadrenergic effects of psychotropic drugs? Addison's disease. High and labile in neuroleptic malignant syndrome, Cushing's syndrome, pain, severe anxiety states
- **Chest**: cardiac heave, evidence of failure (raised jugular venous pressure, peripheral oedema), listen to lung bases, cardiac murmurs, third heart sound. Exclude pleural effusions or any thoracic cage damage. Exclude chest infection
- **Limbs**: tone, power, reflexes. Check arms and legs for injection sites, self-cutting scars, abscesses, wasting, bruising, injures, old fractures, major joint movements. Exclude cellulitis
- **Height and weight:** *Note*: gynaecomastia (neuroleptics, alcohol, other drugs?), body hair distribution (anorexia/pituitary deficit), spider naevi, portocaval anastomoses (? alcohol use). Abdomen – palpate liver edge; constipation due to psychotropics not uncommon; urinary retention due to anticholinergic effects of psychotropics? Possibility of pregnancy? Possibility of urinary tract infection?

If there are any signs or symptoms suggestive of medical illness perform a thorough examination and obtain the necessary physical investigations. Do not prescribe a course of psychotropic drugs.

INVESTIGATIONS

The following are commonly used investigations in psychiatry and should be considered if the clinical history is suggestive of organic illness. They should not be routinely ordered and are most likely to be of value in the elderly.

- **Psychological:** behavioural analysis. Structured instruments to evaluate psychopathology, suicidality and aspects of personality and their response to interventions and over time
- **IQ assessment**: neuropsychological assessment if focal deficits identified or suspected
- **Social**: further assessment of housing, finance, benefits, bus-pass availability, debts, family support, leisure and day care. Social services needs assessment
- **Blood**: full blood count, urea and electrolytes, liver function tests (e.g. γ-glutamyl transferase for liver damage due to alcohol), thyroid function tests, Venereal Disease Research Laboratories test (VDRL) – in special circumstances human immunodeficiency virus (HIV), hepatitis B, hepatitis C, blood alcohol, therapeutic drug monitoring (lithium, carbamazepine, phenytoin) and to check compliance in refractory cases (e.g. antidepressant levels), paracetamol and salicylate levels after overdose
- **Urine**: drug screens, culture and sensitivity for infection, glucose dipsticks, pregnancy tests
- **X-ray**: after trauma or if systemic illness suspected on basis of history and examination: skull, chest, abdomen, limbs – after trauma
- **Computerized tomography and magnetic resonance imaging**: in neuropsychiatric presentations
- **Electroencephalogram**: in neuropsychiatric presentations

SUMMARIZING THE ASSESSMENT: FORMULATION

In view of the considerable amount of information elicited during a full psychiatric assessment, the ability to succinctly summarize this information in order to effectively communicate with colleagues is essential.

DESCRIPTION

- Brief statement about demographics and presentation with 'active problem' list
- Brief statement about relevant past psychiatric history and current treatment
- Brief statement about personal and family history of relevance
- Important mental state findings

DIAGNOSIS

Give the differential diagnoses along with findings in support or contradicting each of these diagnoses.

EXPLANATIONS

Why this patient, why now and why in this manner? Indicate protective and vulnerability factors. Use a grid:

	Biological	Social	Psychological
Precipitating			
Predisposing			
Perpetuating			

ACCURACY AND LIMITATIONS OF ASSESSMENT

- Personality: yours and the patient's
- Communication/rapport
- Other sources of information
- Inconsistencies in account
- Cultural factors: linguistic difficulties, female psychiatrist preferred
- Family assessment

MANAGEMENT

- Present a plan for each of the problems identified
- Present a timescale for implementation and review of each intervention
- Present sources of further information
- Precautions: risk analysis and procedures to prevent suicide and other adverse outcomes
- Engage other agencies: voluntary/statutory, health/social
- List: name of keyworker and individuals involved, their contact addresses and telephone numbers
- List Mental Health Act status: appeals, dates of tribunals, manager's hearings

REFERENCES

1. Gelder MG, Gath D, Mayou R. Oxford textbook of psychiatry. Oxford: Oxford Medical Publications, 1994.
2. Kendall RE, Zeally AK. Companion to psychiatric studies. Edinburgh: Churchill Livingstone, 1995.
3. Sims A. Symptoms in the mind. An introduction to descriptive psychopathology. London: Baillière Tindall, 1988.
4. Ryle A. Cognitive analytic therapy: active participation in change. Chichester: John Wiley & Sons, 1990.
5. Kopelman M. Structured psychiatric interview: assessment of the cognitive state. Br J Hosp Med 1994; 52: 277–281.
6. Lishman WA. Organic psychiatry, 2nd ed. Oxford: Blackwell Scientific, 1987.

7. Folstein MF, Folstein SE, McHugh PR. 'Mini-mental state'. A practical method for grading the cognitive state of patients for the clinician. J Psychiatr Res 1975; 12: 189–198.

SECTION II

Psychiatric Emergencies: a Problem-based Approach

THE ANXIOUS PATIENT

Anxiety is a symptom of many psychiatric disorders, including alcohol withdrawal, but may also be a normal adaptive response to a hostile or threatening environment.

SYMPTOMS

- **IDEATIONAL**
  - Apprehension
  - Fear
- **SOMATIC**
  - Dry mouth, difficulty swallowing
  - Palpitations
  - Flushing
  - Pallor
  - Hyperventilation
  - Tremor
  - Increased gastrointestinal motility
  - Chest pain
  - Backache, headache, fatigue
  - Diarrhoea
  - Urinary frequency
  - Paraesthesia
- **CHRONOLOGICAL**
  - Episodic
  - Continuous
  - Stress-related
- **BEHAVIOURAL**
  - Avoidance
  - Rituals, e.g. checking
  - Startle response heightened
  - Hypervigilance
  - Poor concentration
  - Insomnia
  - Reduced libido

CLINICAL FEATURES

Psychological symptoms

Irritability, difficulty in concentrating (patient complains of poor memory), fearful anticipation, sensitivity to noise, a feeling of restlessness, repetitive worrying thoughts (ruminations). Appearance: strained, furrowed forehead, tense, tremulous, pale and sweating and tearful.

Physical symptoms and signs

Autonomic symptoms (see somatic symptoms above), sleep disturbance, muscular tension, overbreathing, tingling in fingers and perioral paraesthesia due to hyperventilation.

DIFFERENTIAL DIAGNOSIS

Psychiatric

- Schizophrenia
- Mania
- Depression
- Generalized anxiety disorder
- Phobic disorder
- Panic disorder
- Obsessive–compulsive disorder
- Post-traumatic stress disorder
- Acute reaction to stress
- Adjustment reaction

Physical/organic states presenting as an anxiety state

- **Alcohol and drug withdrawal/intoxication**: restlessness, overactivity, disorientation, inability to register information, fearful affect, lability of mood, sweating, tremor, visual hallucinations in delirium tremens (classically small, mobile, coloured animals or insects) associated with paranoia, fits, diarrhoea, abdominal cramps, sensitivity to noise, hyperalgesia. Look for evidence of drug use (injection sites, abscesses, liver flap, tender liver with hepatomegaly). Raised γ-glutamyl transferase or mean corpuscular volume indicates chronic excessive alcohol use. Liver function tests may be deranged in alcohol misuse
- **Dementia**: disorientation, registers information but 5-minute recall impaired (disorder of learning), nominal aphasia, constructional apraxia, often unconcerned with impairments unless cognitive testing culminates in a catastrophic reaction, absence of systemic disease, focal neurological signs may be present in multi-infarct dementia and dementia of Alzheimer's type. A useful clinical picture, the distinction of which from dementia is in question, is that of subcortical dementia distinguished by lack of motivation, affective changes, abnormal gait and posture, dysarthria, ataxia, tremor with a gradual onset in the absence of language, learning and calculating disabilities
- **Thyrotoxicosis**: sweating, heat intolerance, check for goitre, tachycardia, tremor, lid lag and exophthalmos
- **Hypoglycaemia**: hunger, sweating, tremor, fatigue, dizziness, fear and apprehension. Check for a history of diabetes; glucose dipsticks will quickly establish whether intravenous glucose is necessary
- **Unstable angina**
- **Phaeochromocytoma**: episodic sweating, headache, hypertension and

tremor. Rare but life-threatening; episodic anxiety with hypertension; check fundi (normal if episodic hypertension), tachycardia, urine screening test for 4-hydroxy, 3-methoxy mandelic acid (VMA; detects about 85% of cases)

- **Carcinoid syndrome**: episodic hypertension, sweating and flushing. Urinary 5-hydroxyindoleacetic acid (5-HIAA) elevated
- **HIV**: men more than women, risk factors include intravenous drug use, gay and bisexual men and partners
- **Multiple sclerosis**: lability of mood
- **Intracranial tumours**: personality changes accompany these, lability of mood, aggression

IMMEDIATE MANAGEMENT

- The acutely anxious patient will be very distressed. They and their family may insist that you do something
- Ensure that hyperventilation is not due to a chest infection or traumatic chest injury; check the pulse and blood pressure. Hyperventilation can be helped by breathing in and out of a paper bag so as to raise the plasma $P\text{CO}_2$. It is a low plasma $P\text{CO}_2$ that is responsible for light-headedness, dizziness and paraesthesia
- Calm the patient by removal from a busy casualty department to a quieter room. Reassurance and calm explanation that the symptoms are due to the physiological effects of adrenaline (epinephrine) may be sufficient
- Acutely anxious patients may be too distressed to listen and become irritable and terrified
- Oral diazepam (5–10 mg) should be sufficient. If a severe anxiety state with marked motor overactivity, fear or a severe panic attack with loss of control then a slow (1 mg/min) intravenous injection of diazepam (5–10 mg; higher risk of thrombophlebitis with i.v. diazepam) should abate the attack
- Follow this with a discussion of the undesirable effects of benzodiazepines and an explanation and exploration of factors exacerbating the anxiety state. A behavioural treatment programme individually or in groups should be arranged as soon as possible. If this was a single attack it may not happen again
- If panic disorder, social anxiety or generalized anxiety is diagnosed or anxiety is related to agoraphobia or obsessive–compulsive disorder, then the 5-HT reuptake inhibitors (selective serotonin reuptake inhibitors – SSRIs) and venlafaxine have been shown to be of value even in the absence of depressive symptoms. These can take several weeks to become effective (see pp. 225–228). The initial increase in anxiety that sometimes accompanies the prescription of SSRIs responds to the **short-term** prescription of a benzodiazepine
- Avoid prescribing benzodiazepines and inform the GP of any action taken. This group is vulnerable to developing dependence

THE HOSTILE PATIENT

The patient in this situation may be actively violent, threatening violence or have been violent. Violence may be directed at property or people. The aim is to gain control of the situation quickly, assess the aetiological factors involved and treat the patient if necessary.

PREDICTORS OF VIOLENT BEHAVIOUR

- **Recent violent behaviour**
- **Previous violence**: early account in childhood with fights at school, cruelty to pets, exposure to violence in formative years, severe emotional deprivation, imprisonment for violent offences (rape, murder, manslaughter)
- **Carrying weapons**: knives or guns or use in previous incidents
- **Sex**: men are consistently more violent than women
- **Socioeconomic status**: commoner in lower socioeconomic class and if fewer social supports
- **Disinhibiting factors**: drug and alcohol intoxication, organic – head injury, frontal lobe damage; violence less common with temporal lobe damage
- **Impaired ability to reason and deal with frustration**: learning difficulties or psychiatric disorder, command hallucinations, paranoid delusions
- **Aggression in response to psychiatric symptoms**: psychomotor agitation, excitative stage after catatonia, manic excitement
- **Dissocial personality disorder**

DIFFERENTIAL DIAGNOSIS

Psychiatric disorders associated with violence

- Schizophrenia (especially paranoid schizophrenia)
- Mania (manic excited states)
- Depression (agitated)
- Personality disorder: antisocial, borderline, intermittent explosive
- Post-traumatic stress disorder
- Acute reaction to stress

Physical/organic causes

- **Delirium**: violence may occur during a delirious state if the patient is experiencing persecutory or threatening delusions or hallucinations. Look for fluctuating pattern along with altering level of consciousness. Repetitive violence associated with delirium may occur more often at night. Consider head injury; postictal confusional states may also present like this although violence and goal-directed activity is unusual in postictal states. Exclude physical causes of delirium in the elderly (see pp. 31, 76 and 205)
- **Drug and alcohol intoxication or withdrawal**: alcohol acts as a disin-

hibiting agent but alcohol withdrawal may result in delirium tremens. Milder states of withdrawal are characterized by increased sensitivity to noise and irritability. Chronic alcohol use may result in alcoholic dementia or acute encephalopathy due to hepatic failure or thiamine deficiency (Wernicke's encephalopathy). Wernicke's encephalopathy may present in subacute form, so a high index of suspicion is required. Alcoholic hallucinosis and delusional disorder related to alcohol use should be considered. Again, paranoid beliefs and command hallucinations are associated with violence. Withdrawal states related to sedative dependence (benzodiazepines, barbiturates, heroin) result in overactivity and irritability with a lower tolerance of frustration. Acute psychoses may occur with amfetamine, cocaine or LSD use. Violence may occur in a disorganized way as a consequence

- **Dementia**: hallucinations and paranoid beliefs can arise in the demented. Impaired reasoning capacity plus lower threshold for frustration
- **Organic personality disorder**: emotional lability, irritability, outbursts of anger or aggression. Cognitive changes with suspicion. This may involve frontal lobe damage. Abnormal electroencephalogram (EEG) may be present with temporal slowing

IMMEDIATE MANAGEMENT

- Take as many details as you can when the patient is referred, paying particular attention to predictors of violence. Use all sources of information (past notes, etc.) to make a quick assessment of dangerousness. Assess involvement of weapons and potential for violence, most severe and recent offences
- Clear the public and other staff from the area. If patient is armed do not tackle yourself, contact the police and ask them to disarm. Involve hospital security
- Try talking the patient down in a confident but non-confrontational manner. If unsuccessful or if more violence is threatened or ensues proceed to control and restraint techniques
- Secure adequate numbers of experienced staff trained in control and restraint techniques. There should be one person per limb and one for the head. One other member of staff (usually the doctor) to administer medication. Establish clearly who is in charge of the situation
- Use an intramuscular neuroleptic (haloperidol 5–10 mg or droperidol 5 mg). If the patient has been exposed to neuroleptic medication previously, higher doses may be required. Wait 20 minutes and if still necessary repeat the dose. Continue this process until rapid tranquillization is achieved. Use i.v diazepam as an adjunct (10–20 mg; i.v. diazepam is associated with a higher incidence of thrombophlebitis). Flumazenil is an alternative that does not have this problem. If an intravenous line cannot be established, use i.m. lorazepam 2–4 mg (do not use i.m. diazepam as it is erratically absorbed). An alternative to this approach is to use a combination of benzodiazepines and antipsychotic from the outset. This has the advantage that hostility

related to anxiety is more quickly reduced, and the total amount of antipsychotic required is likely to be less

- Once 'made safe', exclude other causes of disturbance such as head injury, delirium (and causes thereof) or substance intoxication. *Note*: if alcoholic delirium tremens is the cause of the behaviour then neuroleptics may precipitate a fit, as they reduce the fit threshold. Nurse individually with frequent measurements of pulse, blood pressure, temperature and neurology
- Consider legal status. A Mental Health Act section for assessment may be indicated. If a clear diagnosis has previously been established and the patient has relapsed then a section 3 is appropriate. If a patient is violent a section is not required before you act. You can proceed under common law as you are acting in the best interests of the patient and the public
- If an open ward is unsafe (for patients, staff or the public if patient absconds) then a locked ward or forensic unit may be required. Discuss this during a debriefing session with all the staff involved

THE DEPRESSED PATIENT

A patient may complain specifically of depression but only about 20% of primary-care attenders actually exhibit their distress in this way. It is more likely that the clinician considers the patient to be depressed and then evaluates other possible explanations so as to guide treatment choices. Careful assessment is necessary in order to elicit the symptoms and signs of depression.

SYMPTOMS AND SIGNS

PHYSICAL SYMPTOMS
Lack of energy, sleeplessness, aches and pain

MOOD AND FEELING STATES
Fed up, bored, angry or irritable, anxious, panicky feelings, tension

BEHAVIOUR
Avoid going out, self-neglect, not hungry, not eating and losing weight, checking compulsively (e.g. light switches are off, doors locked etc.), inactivity, including sitting still for hours (may be stupor)

THOUGHTS – DELUSIONAL
Of being punished, of wrongdoing, of committing terrible crimes, of rotting insides, of having no body

THOUGHTS – MORBID
Of something dreadful about to happen, nothing to look forward to, of

harm coming to self or family unless patient behaves in a certain way. Unable to stop worries

- **THOUGHTS – SUICIDAL**
  Wants to die, has tried to hurt self, has tried to kill self, has plans to kill self. Worry about bodily functions. Feeling worthless and of no value to anyone

- **OTHER CORE SYMPTOMS**
  Poor memory, concentration and learning skills. Loss of interest in usual hobbies

DIFFERENTIAL DIAGNOSIS

Psychiatric

- Major depressive episode
- Minor depressive episode
- Generalized anxiety disorder
- Obsessive–compulsive disorder
- Panic disorder
- Puerperal states: psychosis and depression
- Agoraphobia

Organic

- Alcohol or substance misuse
- **Infectious disease**: HIV, pneumonia, influenza, syphilis
- **Endocrine disorder**: Cushing's syndrome, thyroid disorder
- **Neoplastic**: pancreas, lung, cerebral
- **Iatrogenic**: prescribed medication
- **Neuropsychiatric**: dementia, epilepsy, stroke

IMMEDIATE MANAGEMENT

- The priority is to evaluate the degree of depression, the presence of suicidal thoughts and intent and the selection of the appropriate package of interventions. The interview should be carried out in a comfortable environment. Relatives often wish to be present while the patient is being assessed. This is usually fine but may prevent the patient from expressing their true feelings; preferably some time should be set aside to see the relatives separately. A selective physical examination will be of value if the history and specific symptoms are suggestive of an organic component
- Depressed patients often take longer to think through and respond to questions put to them. Allow answers to emerge. Do not pressure the patient into responding. They will be unable to respond openly if a trusting relationship has not been established. Silences are often more uncomfortable for the clinician, who may have other patients

to see. A silence for the depressed patient will give them the time to convey much of how they are feeling

- In the presence of suicidality the extent of it should be assessed in detail (see below and p. 49). If the patient is depressed and suicidal or at risk of serious self-harm, admit them for assessment. Night sedation is necessary if there are overt symptoms of anxiety and agitation. If possible and usually in the absence of an immediate threat to life the option of a return home under the supervision of a friend or relative may be arranged as long as the depressive symptoms are **actively managed**. Involve the patient's GP and make an outpatient appointment for the patient to see the psychiatrist
- Sending a patient home with antidepressants without a proper assessment of suicide risk, or arrangements to monitor depressive symptoms at least weekly in the early stages, may lead to a completed suicide. If there are social indicators of higher suicide risk, avoid sedative antidepressants. Use one of the selective 5-HT reuptake inhibitors (SSRIs), which are less dangerous in overdose
- Interventions directed at social and psychological factors in the aetiology and maintenance of depression should be identified and offered to the patient, e.g. improved housing, refuge for victims of violence, etc. Involve the duty social worker early. Specific depressive beliefs, including contemplating suicide, are amenable to cognitive therapy. This skill can be exercised in the emergency situation to (1) identify depressogenic beliefs that can later be targeted by cognitive therapy, (2) evaluate the fixity of the beliefs, (3) shift the target beliefs (suicidal thoughts) as part of acute treatment and assessment

THE SUICIDAL PATIENT

Suicidality refers to deliberate and potentially fatal acts of self-harm. Suicidal thoughts are part of depressive symptomatology but can arise in many psychiatric disorders and should be specifically enquired about during assessment. The exact thoughts, feelings and actions of the patient must be identified and recorded in as much detail as possible.

SYMPTOMS AND SIGNS

MOVEMENTS – DEPRESSIVE

Psychomotor retardation, stupor, absence of reactivity of expression. Agitation, irritability, impulsive behaviour with or without violence to property or other people

MOVEMENTS – MANIC

Consider manic excitement as part of a mixed affective state

- **THOUGHTS – DEPRESSIVE**
  Slowing or absence of any thinking. Worthlessness, hopelessness, helplessness, wish to escape from torment, wish to join dead relatives, wish to die as the most suitable punishment, wish to die as the only solution to social and relationship problems, wish to die for no obvious identifiable reason. May be accompanied by wish for punishment and guilt, of wrongdoing, of complete poverty (financial or physical, e.g. 'I have no heart' as part of nihilistic delusions)
- **THOUGHTS – PSYCHOTIC**
  Delusions of immortality/being God and therefore able to be reborn, of taking one's life before persecutors (the devil, MI5, neighbours, etc.) do so
- **SEVERITY INDICATORS:**
  - Evidence of careful planning
  - Previous attempts
  - Psychiatric diagnosis – recent visit to GP or psychiatrist
  - Chronic physical illness (pain, terminal illness)
  - Serious attempt
  - Violent method chosen
  - Family history of psychiatric disorder
  - Social/life events – bereavement, unemployment
  - Male
  - Elderly (rising incidence in young men and young Asian women)
  - Single
  - No support networks

CLINICAL FEATURES

Deliberate self-harm: repeated acts of non-fatal self-harm with no intention to die must be distinguished and can arise as part of acute distress states (bereavement, separation from partner, end of a relationship, social stressors) or from persistent conditions such as anxiety states, eating disorders, personality disorders and depressive states in schizophrenia or manic depressive illness. Affective symptoms can occur in isolation or as part of these syndromes. Alcohol use is common around the time of deliberate self harm or a suicide attempt.

DIFFERENTIAL DIAGNOSIS AND ASSOCIATED DISORDERS

Psychiatric

- Affective disorder (including bipolar)
- Schizophrenia
- Persistent anxiety states
- Personality disorder
- Dual diagnoses: any of above with substance abuse

Organic

- **Alcoholism**: associated depression and social problems

- **Substance misuse**: social adversity, homelessness, financial problems, unbearable withdrawal symptoms
- **Epilepsy**: persistent
- **Chronic disabling physical illness**: loss of limbs, nervous system disorder
- **Chronic pain**
- **Terminal illness**: cancer

IMMEDIATE MANAGEMENT

- If the patient has taken an overdose or there is an open wound requiring immediate attention after self-injury, ensure that this is attended to first. If another team (medical or surgical) take over the immediate care ensure that they are fully aware of the suicidal potential and that the patient is adequately emotionally supported and supervised before a detailed assessment can be carried out
- If the patient is refusing life-saving treatment, explain carefully the risks of not having treatment, detail the consequences and the timescale for them to take place, and explain the impact of treatment immediately or of delayed treatment. Evaluate the patient's *capacity* to make an informed decision: they must understand the nature and consequences of their choice and *you* must be satisfied that they are able to appraise the information put before them. Record your assessment of capacity. If they do not have the capacity to make an informed choice, treat under common law. Physical treatments cannot be sanctioned by placement on a detention order under the Mental Health Act, unless a physical disorder is contributing or solely responsible for an altered mental state. If the patient is trying to leave or is likely to injure themselves again, or has harmed themselves, they should be detained to complete an assessment (pp. 57 and 69)
- Until this is enacted it is essential that the patient be detained in their own best interests. In this situation clearly identify which nursing team (accident and emergency, ward) will be providing continuing supervision (24 hours)
- Involve and inform family members. They may be invaluable in helping persuade the patient to receive treatment. If the patient has not taken an overdose and has not harmed themselves, assess their immediate suicidal intent
- Interview: establish rapport. Do not be afraid about asking questions about suicide:
  - Do they still want to die?
  - What are their thoughts about the failed attempt?
  - Are they likely to do this again?
  - Do they have a detailed plan?
  - Is the chosen method lethal?
  - Did they allow for the possibility of being saved?
  - Will they have the opportunity to enact the plan?
  - Have the precipitating circumstances been resolved?

- Had they organized all their affairs in anticipation of a completed suicide?
- Was depression recently diagnosed?
- Were they prescribed some medication?
- What other interventions have been tried?
- Were any specific interventions helpful?
- Who will they go to for help?
- Will they see their GP?
- Following discharge what measures are in place to prevent a recurrence of depression and suicidal acts?
- Would they consider continued drug treatment, psychotherapy or maintenance electroconvulsive therapy (ECT)?

- If the *risks remain high* and there are no community interventions available or acceptable to the patient, consider admission. If there are clear signs of depression (see pp. 154–161) or social factors that are not immediately remedied, consider admission either for the safe treatment of depression in a protected environment under supervision or to intervene in the crisis
- Admission under a section of the Mental Health Act may be especially necessary if (1) the patient expresses inconsistent views about their wish to remain voluntarily or return home, (2) there is a high likelihood of absconding, (3) there is the possibility of a fatal suicide attempt
- Agree the observation requirements to the nursing staff. Once on the ward ensure that the patient is adequately supervised, and record the level of observations necessary after a consensus is agreed with the nursing staff. If the patient is depressed but does not need admission, this finding will be the conclusion of a careful assessment that determines that the patient is not acutely suicidal or that their suicidality has abated as a result of social and psychological interventions delivered there and then, e.g. arrangements for accommodation, help with financial problems, providing further support by telephone availability and an outpatient appointment or home visit
- Beware: denial of suicidal intent, impulsive distress, anger, malignant alienation, assumptions of improvement in the absence of evidence, poorly planned and coordinated treatment regimens[1] and repeated self-harm[2]

THE PERSONALITY DISORDERED PATIENT: A CAUTIONARY NOTE

The diagnosis of personality disorder is a difficult one to make on one interview (see pp. 174–180). The term is used widely by professionals and the public, but often inaccurately. This section aims to identify the types of presentation in which personality disorder is the predominant factor; however, it is most likely to occur as a secondary diagnosis to other psychiatric conditions. A corroborative history is required before making a definitive diagnosis.

CLINICAL PRESENTATIONS

- **Aggression to staff or public**
- **Demanding prescriptions – for self or to market on the street**
- **After street brawl**
- **Intoxicated – withdrawal states**
- **Homelessness and demands for housing yet not taking up offers of what is available**
- **Threats of self-harm – actual self-harm as a public display**
- **Accusations of abandonment by services, family, partners**
- **Presenting in crisis yet not accepting help or not adhering to any structured plan**
- **Partners or children are presented – Munchausen syndrome**
- **Presents with physical symptoms in order to enter the sick role**
- **Brought by police**
- **Criminality – opinion sought urgently**

MAKING THE RIGHT DECISION

You cannot ignore this population. The fact that some patients are unpleasant can influence your judgement in favour of dismissing them. These presentations can arise from a diverse number of distinct disorders, ranging from depression through schizophrenia to pure dissocial personality disorder and criminality. People with a personality disorder have a higher risk than the general public of suicide and in view of their inability to maintain successful relationships or social circumstance are likely to develop psychiatric disorders. Patients in distress may act in a manner that recruits from onlookers the label of personality disorder. Distressed people may behave in maladaptive ways and their coping strategies become more extreme. A crisis ensues when their strategies are increasingly unsuccessful.

Careful assessment, with information from relatives and friends as well as past health and social service contacts, is essential. If these people or agencies cannot be contacted immediately, make another time to meet with the patient, explaining the need to obtain as much information as possible. This is especially important in instances where prescriptions for controlled drugs are being sought. Always discuss your assessment with a senior colleague and record your concerns and the reasoning behind your conclusions and management plan.

Where there is sufficient information to make a diagnosis of personality disorder or where the demands of the patient are escalating and unreasonable making such a diagnosis more likely, *consider the possibility of a psychiatric disorder, the risk of suicide and violence to others*. If after an assessment meeting there is no evidence of a psychiatric disorder, admission is contraindicated. It will only reinforce maladaptive illness behaviour. Make it clear that, although admission is not deemed necessary, you will secure help in any other way and arrange for the patient to be seen again. If there are any potential social interventions that can be arranged, do so. This may involve urgent liaison with social services or a referral. Psychotherapy should be considered and if the patient is agreeable an assessment session for suitability should be booked as soon as possible.

Where the patient is complaining of physical illness and yet there are obvious signs of personality disorder, do a physical examination or arrange for the medical team or Accident & Emergency staff to review the patient, depending on level of urgency. If the history or presentation does not make sense or is incomplete and there remains a risk of self-harm or of serious physical illness as yet undetected, an admission for assessment will be necessary. This should be arranged after *careful discussion with nursing staff and the consultant*. If there are any concerns about violence or substance misuse while on the ward an admission contract may prevent the matter arising in crisis. Think of all the possible problems that might arise and record a management plan for each.

ASSESSMENT CHECKLIST

- **Psychiatric disorder?**
- **Physical illness?**
- **Substance misuse?**
- **Violence potential?**
- **Acting out potential if admitted?**
- **Psychotherapeutic interventions?**
- **Any success experiences: work, hobbies?**
- **Intelligence and ability to tolerate frustration?**
- **Suicide risk?**
- **Any meaningful relationships?**
- **Previous interventions (especially failed ones)**
- **Management plan: disseminate to colleagues**

THE HALLUCINATING PATIENT

Hallucinations are perceptions in the absence of a stimulus and can arise in any modality. The commonest are auditory, visual and somatic hallucinations. True hallucinations appear to arise in external space and have the quality of a perception following a stimulus. The prevalence and significance of hallucinations appears to vary across cultures.

SYMPTOMS AND SIGNS

- AUDITORY
  - Distractibility, inaccessibility, incongruent affect
  - Sudden changes of mood – fear, elation, giggling
  - Sudden changes of posture as if listening
  - Requests for silence
  - Holding a conversation with voices – whispering to self
  - Inability to think clearly
  - Occasionally no evidence of voices – disclosure after assessment
  - In second or third person, command or commenting
- VISUAL
  - Looking into corners of the room
  - Sudden changes in affect – pleasure to terror, fear and depression
  - Usually associated in organic conditions with clouding of consciousness
  - Pulling at clothes or objects
  - Inability to get attention (usually with delirium)
  - Of people, faces, animals, scenes (fires of hell and the devil)

  Note: people with little sight can hallucinate visually
- SOMATIC
  - Sensations can arise in any part of the body – mouth, head, genitals; attribution of sensations to passers-by can lead to assaults

CLINICAL FEATURES

Distinguish visual hallucinations from eidetic imagery, when patients can voluntarily generate scenes that are vivid. Otherwise, imagery is less vivid and has the quality of not being real. Dim lighting potentiates illusion formation: emergence of images out of shapes, colours, taking the form of real objects. Visual hallucinations more commonly arise in organic states. Auditory hallucinations may also arise in organic states but in this instance the voices are fragmented and transitory; other signs of organic states help distinguish psychiatric states from organic ones. Distinguish from pseudohallucinations, in which the perception is not as real and seems to arise from within the person. Pseudohallucinations are usually ego-syntonic, whereas true hallucinations are usually ego-dystonic. Hallucinatory experiences can fall within the realm of culturally sanctioned phenomena and hence are not always a sign of illness.

Discussion with the patient's cultural reference groups will highlight if the experience is culturally inconsistent with health.

DIFFERENTIAL DIAGNOSIS

Psychiatric

- Schizophrenia
- Major affective disorder: depression or mania with psychosis
- Brief psychoses and dissociative disorders
- Puerperal psychoses

Organic

- Alcoholic hallucinosis, alcohol withdrawal (delirium tremens) and drug intoxication withdrawal (stimulants are more likely to produce this)
- Dementia
- Delirium and metabolic disorders
- Temporal lobe epilepsy
- Tumours (CNS)
- Eye or retinal disease

IMMEDIATE MANAGEMENT

- The management of the hallucinating patient should focus on the exclusion of an organic disorder (see pp. 32, 202–203 and 206). Those with unexplained visual hallucinations should have an assessment of their visual fields and an ophthalmological examination. Pre-existing eye disease may contribute to the development of visual phenomena. Similarly the hard of hearing may have auditory hallucinations and middle ear disease should be excluded, especially if the presentation is atypical. The assessment aims to make a confident psychiatric diagnosis and management plan on the basis of a history and psychopathology
- Patients may be frightened and agitated. Poorly lit, noisy areas may exacerbate their fear. Remove the patient to a calm environment. Engage them in conversation and examine to what extent their functioning is impaired by hallucinations. During the course of a conversation signs and symptoms might spontaneously arise. Detailed questions about hallucinations are unlikely to result in immediate answers and it may take time to enable the patient to feel comfortable. Allaying some of their fear may be a necessary prerequisite. There is often a conviction among staff that some patients are hearing voices but on direct questioning they will deny it
- Identify which of the features above are present and support the view that the patient is hallucinating. Some patients with persistent symptoms and in continuing contact with psychiatric services do not

wish anyone to know of their hallucinations for fear of enforced treatment. Others may not be able to disentangle specific hallucinations from their range of abnormal experience. This assessment is made especially complex in individuals who have a limited pre-morbid capacity for communication: those with learning difficulties, head injuries, children, stroke victims, partially sighted, hard of hearing, etc.

- The management of individual patients is that of the primary diagnosis. Neuroleptic medication is of value in both organic and non-organic hallucinations. Generalized anxiety-relieving measures, as discussed on p. 16, are of value in the acute situation. If anxiety is very prominent a benzodiazepine (diazepam 5–10 mg p.o.) should be given in addition to a neuroleptic (haloperidol 5–10 mg p.o.); if sedation is required use 50–200 mg chlorpromazine, depending on body mass of patient (monitor blood pressure). If the patient is acutely disturbed and effective communication cannot be established then enforced sedation will be necessary (see pp. 18 and 19)
- If the presentation is atypical and there are difficulties with obtaining a complete assessment (different culture, deaf, learning difficulties), avoid neuroleptics and any other medication if possible until a full assessment as an inpatient is completed

THE PARANOID PATIENT

The term 'paranoid' is loosely applied to those who feel persecuted but in a psychiatric sense refers also to presentations of which the content is self-referential. A variety of self-referential symptoms can arise in the context of many of the major psychiatric disorders as well as a range of organic states.

SYMPTOMS AND SIGNS

PERSECUTORY DELUSIONS

Neighbours, strangers, family members either torment or are watching or are responsible for a series of adverse events. Organizations or large institutions (real or delusory) may be held responsible for the patient's distress

PERSECUTORY HALLUCINATIONS

Influence the content of delusional beliefs: 'we'll kill you … we will get you … you did it'

GRANDIOSE DELUSIONS

Having a special skill, role or mission in the world, especially when there are elaborate beliefs about why the patient was chosen

MORBID JEALOUSY

Conviction that partner is having affair – checks partner's clothes, movements. Denial is interpreted as proof but if through frustration a confession is made, this only leads to exacerbation of the mental disturbance. Patients are potentially dangerous as they may resort to violence. Morbid jealousy is associated with alcoholism and is commoner in men. It can arise in organic states

EROTOMANIA

Typical account is of a woman who falls in love with an unattainable man of higher status. All acts by the man are interpreted to be consistent with his love being returned to her. Actions by the object of adoration, even if openly discouraging or bluntly negative, are interpreted as signals of the person's true but discreet love for the patient

SHARED DELUSIONS

When two people present with an unusual story it is often adopted as reality but in cases of induced psychoses two or more people living in isolation from others can develop a shared delusional belief that is self-referential and/or persecutory. In 90% of instances those sharing the belief are family members (sisters are commonest, followed by husband and wife, mother and child, two brothers, brother and sister, father and child, and unrelated)

SENSITIVE PERSONALITY TRAITS

In personality-disordered – sense of injustice and prejudice, sensitive to any potential criticism. It may be difficult to distinguish severe paranoid personality disorder from paranoid psychoses

DIFFERENTIAL DIAGNOSIS

Psychiatric

- Schizophrenia
- Affective psychoses: persecutory and self-referential symptoms
- Paranoid personality disorder
- Borderline states
- Severe acute distress: brief reactive psychoses
- Induced psychoses: may be persecutory
- Morbid jealousy (Othello syndrome): more self-referential than persecutory
- Erotomania (de Clérambault's syndrome): self-referential

Organic

- Drug-induced states: alcohol withdrawal (delirium tremens), cocaine
- Dementia
- Delirium

IMMEDIATE MANAGEMENT

- The background history is essential, as the patient often appears to be able to hold brief conversations without obvious evidence of abnormality. Only when the specifics of their beliefs are examined, along with accounts from third parties, does the true picture emerge. This is why shared delusions are especially difficult to identify
- The cultural context of beliefs should also be understood, or at least evaluated, by recruiting someone from the same culture before labelling beliefs as delusional. Substance misuse and organic conditions must be excluded
- Bizarre, mood-incongruent beliefs and hallucinations are likely to suggest schizophrenia, whereas mood-congruent symptoms are more suggestive of affective psychoses (see p. 154). Brief reactive psychoses arise suddenly and often have an admixture of affective as well as confusional symptoms
- If a diagnosis of affective psychosis or schizophrenia is made, neuroleptic medication will have a role to play in the acute management of distress and disturbance. If, however, the diagnosis includes one of the self-referential and more unusual disorders, the prognosis is poor and separation from the object of the patient's belief or (in the case of shared delusions) from the sharer is the only safe treatment. With Othello and de Clérambault's syndromes there is a risk of violence by the dissatisfied patient. Love turns into grief and may become irritability and anger. Advise the object of attention that immediate separation is necessary and possibly an injunction; advise of the dangers of not doing so and of there being no immediate treatment

THE CONFUSED PATIENT

Confusion refers to objective signs and subjective symptoms suggestive of impaired ability to think clearly. It is not itself diagnostic but raises the possibility of specific organic and non-organic disorders.

SYMPTOMS AND CLINICAL FEATURES

See Table 1 overleaf.

DIFFERENTIAL DIAGNOSIS

Psychiatric

- Schizophrenia
- Brief reactive psychoses

Table 1: Symptoms and clinical features of confusion

Diagnosis	Delirium	Dementia	Non-organic
History	Sudden onset	Insidious	Either
Duration	Short (days)	Long (months)	Either
Consciousness level	Impaired	Normal	Either
Course	Fluctuates	Progressive	Either
Disorientation	++ → +++	+ → +++	Either
Impaired registration	+++	0 → +	0 → +
Affect	Terrified Anxious Irritable	Indifferent Labile	Elated/depressive Labile/terrified
Psychomotor	Poverty Overactivity	Normal	Either
Sleep	++ → +++	0 → ++	Either
Reversibility	Often	Rarely	Often
Poor memory			
Short-term memory impairment	Not testable	+++	0 → +
Long-term memory impairment	Not testable	+ → ++	0
Speech	Rambling/ incoherent	Aphasia	Formal thought disorder, flight of ideas, mute Depressive content Anxiety
Focal neurology	0 → ++	0 → +	0
Focal cognitive signs	0	+ → +++	0

- Depression (pseudodementia)
- Severe anxiety
- Dissociative state (fugue/conversion symptoms)
- Ganser's syndrome
- Munchausen syndrome

Organic

- Delirium – physical illness or alcohol withdrawal (see pp. 76 and 134)
- Dementia (see p. 199)
- Space-occupying lesions
- Epilepsy (simple or complex partial seizures or postictal confusion)

IMMEDIATE MANAGEMENT

- This will largely depend on whether the cause of confusion is delirium, dementia or a non-organic disorder. Exclude an organic cause. Delirium can be a sign of a medical emergency. Delirious patients may be hallucinating and expressing unusual beliefs that can be mistaken for frank psychosis. The fragmentary and transient nature of the symptoms, along with poor registration, would support such a diagnosis. Information is often difficult to elicit and corroborate
- Management should be directed by physical examination and history but will often include obtaining information from an informant about past physical and psychiatric disorders and existing medication, and checking full blood count, urea and electrolytes, liver function tests, glucose, thyroid function tests, B_{12} and folate. Also consider a drug screen, chest X-ray, electrocardiogram (ECG), EEG and computerized tomography (CT) scan. Blood cultures and lumbar puncture are indicated if there is an unexplained temperature or fluctuating consciousness level indicating a possible cerebral infection
- If a dementia is suspected an informant history is invaluable but a good cognitive assessment looking for focal deficits will help formulate a correct diagnosis. Lewy body dementia may present with recurrent delirious episodes. Focal neurology or seizures are suggestive of Alzheimer's disease. Lability of mood and disinhibition may be present in Pick's disease or any frontal lobe pathology. Reversible causes of dementia should be excluded. Immediate management may be directed to assessing the causes of socially embarrassing or hostile behaviour or dealing with immediate accommodation. People who have a dementia are more likely to present with delirium because of concurrent physical illness
- The non-organic disorders include apparent memory impairment due to poor concentration accompanied by psychosis, severe anxiety or acute distress
- Brief reactive psychosis, especially among certain cultural groups, may involve an apparent change in consciousness level. Such states are of short duration and may resolve with supportive counselling, psychotherapy and/or benzodiazepines (rather than neuroleptics). Dissociative states are especially difficult to assess in view of the conspicuous absence of any form of personal identification or informant. A small proportion of people presenting with apparent loss of memory may be ultimately diagnosed as having hospital addiction (Munchausen syndrome) or a Ganser's-syndrome-like state (somatic conversion symptoms, approximate answers, clouding of consciousness and pseudohallucinations). The degree of conscious motivation is the subject of much debate and should be considered after a comprehensive assessment with as much corroborated information as possible

- If the non-organic diagnosis remains uncertain, do not medicate, and assess for symptoms of physical and psychiatric illness, ability to have needs met, ability to interact with other patients and staff and ability to concentrate. Ensure that neurological and cardiorespiratory observations and drug screen and sleep chart are completed. If a dissociative mechanism is suspected then abreaction, once established on a ward, will be the treatment of choice
- If there is a risk of deliberate self-harm or unpredictable behaviour, ensure that adequate supervision is available, with emergency medication if necessary (see pp. 17–24, 213). Consider legal status: if unable to give informed consent and a mental illness is suspected then an assessment for a Mental Health Act section should be arranged. If physical illness is significant then assessment and treatment should be carried out under common law, with a clear documented assessment of competency to give consent to treatment

THE POLICE-ESCORTED PATIENT

The police, in accord with Health Circular 66/90, are encouraged to divert the mentally ill to hospital at an early stage. They may accompany an individual because there is a history of mental illness or of suspected mental illness, or because the individual has sustained significant physical injuries. A psychiatric assessment may be requested by the casualty officer. Domestic violence may be a factor.

SYMPTOMS AND CLINICAL SIGNS

VIOLENCE

Note: Section 136; has patient been charged; offence details; handcuffs necessary? struggling? how many police officers? physical injury sustained by patient and police? accompanying threats of assault or actual assault; nature of inflicted injury or property damage; method used (physical aggression with hands, weapon used, fire involved); ability to hold a conversation calmly; staring with fixed eye contact; invasion of personal space

PSYCHOSIS OR ODD UNEXPLAINED BEHAVIOUR

Hallucinations: distractible, unpredictable, sudden activity, inaccessible periods, second-person command hallucinations, persecutory hallucinations. Delusions: grandiose and omnipotent; are actions based on delusional role? Persecuted with fearfulness and escape behaviours

INTOXICATION OR WITHDRAWAL

Alcohol on breath, disinhibited, fits, blackouts, delirium tremens, dysarthric, needle marks, pupil size, pulse rate, charge involves handling substances

SUICIDE ATTEMPT
Ask the following questions: Where was patient picked up? Caught about to jump off a bridge? Wandering into traffic, on railways lines or the underground? Having inflicted injury on themselves in a public place? Following report of self-injury? Aggression? Why were ambulance staff unable to bring patient? Drowsy but with obvious account of self-harm or evidence of self-injury. Cuts on arms, neck, abdomen, genitals, etc. Bottles of psychotropic and other drugs found when picked up

HOMELESS
Homelessness may compound other problems. It may be the reason for self-harm, fearfulness, or it may have followed a mental illness with a gradual decline in self-care skills; hygiene, clothes appropriate for weather, nutrition, chest infection or tuberculosis?

UNRESPONSIVE
Consider fugue and stupor. Found wandering; personal identifications absent, not responding to questions, mute or withdrawn. Amnesia

DIFFERENTIAL DIAGNOSIS

Psychiatric

- Schizophrenia: first episode or relapse
- Paranoid psychosis
- Bipolar affective disorder: depressive episode (synonym: major depression)
- Bipolar affective disorder: manic episode
- Personality disorder
- Dementia
- Fugue
- Learning difficulties

Organic

- Alcohol intoxication/withdrawal
- Other intoxicated or withdrawal states
- Delirium
- Head injury
- Postictal

IMMEDIATE MANAGEMENT

- The police should contact the duty psychiatrist and the approved social worker (ASW) as soon as they place anyone on a section 136. Alert casualty staff, and the person responsible for identifying a bed should the patient need admission. On arrival check the legal status – section 136 or 135 or informal. The ASW should see the patient whether detained or not. If there are grounds for detention it is good practice to implement a section for admission (section 2 or 3) as soon as possible rather than admit a patient on a section 136. Two section-12-approved doctors need to be sought (or the patient's GP and one section-12-approved doctor; see pp. 57–70). As soon as you have satisfied yourself of the need for formal admission, ensure that the doctors and ASW are aware and identify when they will do a joint assessment. If the patient is to be admitted informally then the section 136 ends once the ASW has assessed the patient. Obtain as much information as possible from the police about any offence and the circumstances of their involvement. If charges are to be dropped then ask the police to remain with the patient until your assessment of dangerousness is complete. You may have to ask for assistance from hospital security

- Ensure that any obvious or severe injuries requiring immediate attention are addressed by the casualty team. Ensure that the staff and assessment environment are safe. If in doubt ask for nursing staff or the police to remain with you during the assessment. Similarly before asking for handcuffs to be removed ensure that the assessment room is comfortable, alarmed and will prevent absconding. Document the time at which each stage of the assessment is completed
- Before the assessment of the patient quickly review past records and consider dangerousness, suicide risk, most recent mental state assessment, identified team providing care, previous treatments and reasons for relapse. Identify past criminal record, psychiatric history, substance misuse history, past incidents of violence and any physical illness
- **The assessment**: learning difficulties and ability to communicate effectively, current suicide intent and most recent attempt, nature of offence, weapons used, intention to harm others, reasons for harming self or others (based on delusional beliefs or in response to hallucinations). Specific psychopathology that may help narrow the differential diagnosis. A cognitive assessment performed at this stage may be invaluable should subsequent court reports be required but is also essential to exclude dementia and may allude to the possibility of a fugue state. Document the patient's detailed account of events and especially their reasons for committing the offence, paying attention to ability to recall details of the event, bizarre explanations, illogical answers, remorse, regret, frequency of carrying weapons, competency to give consent for any treatment offered. The reason given for behaviour leading up to and after the offence warrants careful scrutiny and if unusual or suggestive of mental illness an assessment admission should be recommended. Homelessness may be a factor and should there be no grounds for detention the ASW should assist in temporary placement. Corroborate as much of the personal details as possible with other informants, family, probation officers, relevant carers and psychiatric teams

- Should there be no evidence of mental illness or suicide risk, a personality disorder should be considered, or malingering to avoid prosecution. It is advisable to always discuss the situation with a senior colleague before discharging any patient home off a section 136. Some hospitals insist that only a section-12-approved doctor may recommend this course of action
- Sedation to minimize any immediate threat of violence may be administered under common law. The initial assessment may be impossible because of the threat of violence and the patient must be 'made safe' first. Make detailed notes documenting the times of any incidents, injuries and medication given. Discuss the level of security needed for admission to be safe (locked ward, open ward, forensic unit). Ensure that the ward has adequate staff to supervise such a patient and anticipate problems that may arise. Clarify pass status and ensure that sufficient medication is written up in case an emergency arises or p.r.n. medication is required. Document a clear management plan. If at all possible, when the diagnosis is uncertain (section 2), assess patient without medication unless this would add to the risk of violence or self-harm

THE UNRESPONSIVE PATIENT

SYMPTOMS AND CLINICAL FEATURES

- **Stupor is defined as mutism and akinesis: patient appears alert because of eye movements but is unable to initiate speech or action**
- **Clouding of consciousness**
- **Speech usually absent (minimal)**
- **Eyes move as if awake and may follow an object; if closed, may resist passive eye opening**
- **Diminished attention span for environmental stimuli**
- **If speech intact, amnesia for personal historical details and identity suggests psychogenic amnesia or fugue state or multiple personality disorder**
- **Anxiety symptoms usually absent**
- **Poor memory of events during stupor**
- **Stable respiration, pulse and blood pressure**
- **No neurological signs**
  Look for signs of head injury, pupillary reaction to light, pupillary symmetry, corneal reflex intact; look for focal signs, localizing cranial nerve lesions, fluctuating conscious level, neck stiffness. Consider the possibility

of conversion symptoms if neurological examination and investigations are normal (lumbar puncture, CT/MRI, EEG, glucose, urea and electrolytes, thyroid function tests, liver function tests, follicle-stimulating hormone (FSH), luteinizing hormone (LH), adrenocorticotrophic hormone (ACTH), cortisol, paracetamol, aspirin, alcohol)

DIFFERENTIAL DIAGNOSIS

Psychiatric

- **Schizophrenia**: catatonic states, parkinsonian state, neuroleptic malignant syndrome
- **Affective psychoses**: psychomotor retardation, manic or depressive stupor
- **Dissociative states**: fugue, psychogenic amnesia, multiple personality disorder
- Malingering/Munchausen syndrome

Organic

- **Delirium**: consider all the causes paying special attention to closed head injury, postictal, electrolyte or endocrine imbalance, space-occupying CNS lesion
- **Organic brain disorders**: encephalitis or meningitis
- **Cerebrovascular accidents**: especially bilateral events
- **Drug-induced states**: phencyclidine (PCP), 'crack', solvents, alcohol intoxication

IMMEDIATE MANAGEMENT

- Ensure that there is no evidence of a life-threatening acute brain syndrome. Exclude the possibility of drug-induced state, neuroleptic malignant syndrome or suicide attempt. Ensure that temperature, cardiovascular, respiratory and neurological observations are stable
- Take samples for plasma glucose and chemistry as well as for full blood count and endocrine studies; urine dipsticks for blood, ketones and protein; urinary drug screen; immediately check for plasma glucose using glucose dipsticks. If evidence of muscular rigidity obtain a plasma creatinine phosphokinase (CPK)
- Do a full neurological examination including fundi, reflexes and pupillary size and reaction to light; look for parkinsonian symptoms (drug induced); muscular rigidity, labile temperature and blood pressure, raised CPK, raised white count, myoglobinuria and delirium suggest neuroleptic malignant syndrome
- Obtain an urgent neurological opinion and obtain a magnetic resonance imaging (MRI) scan and EEG, chest X-ray and ECG if indicated clinically

- Use Glasgow Coma Scale to score degree of impairment of consciousness
- Examine any past records and obtain informant history; those with psychogenic stupor, amnesia or fugue states often have no personal details or contacts through which to corroborate their account. Verify suicide risk factors, past history of major mental illness and effective treatments as well as recent contact with services
- If a diagnosis of psychogenic stupor is favoured, consider adequate physical care while symptoms are so disabling, e.g. pressure sores, hydration, concomitant physical illness, urinary retention
- Abreaction and hypnosis may be part of subsequent plan but if immobility is life-threatening and major affective psychosis or catatonia has not been excluded, ECT should be considered as an emergency
- Consider legal status of patient and whether best managed on medical or psychiatric ward. Common law allows emergency treatment. If evidence of mental illness or suicide risk assess for formal admission for treatment

THE SEXUALLY DISINHIBITED PATIENT

Sexually disinhibited behaviour may be a manifestation of psychiatric disorder, organic disease or personality organization; it may be goal-directed or disorganized; behaviours that would be acceptable privately may be displayed in a public place. The police may become involved if a public offence is committed.

SYMPTOMS AND CLINICAL SIGNS

- **EXPOSURE OF GENITALS**
  - Erect penis suggests aggression, flaccid penis suggests inadequacy
  - Masturbation in public
- **GENITAL SELF-MUTILATION**
  Guilt, depression, acting on bizarre delusions
- **Presence of specific sexual dysfunction or marital problems**
- **PSYCHOSEXUAL HISTORY**
  Experience of relationships, successes and failures
- **EXPERIENCE OF ABUSE OR RAPE**
  Sexualized behaviour in children, or less commonly in adults, may indicate sexual trauma
- **PREFERRED SEXUAL OBJECT**
  Fetishes

- **FORENSIC HISTORY**
  Violent, sexual and other offences
- **CLOTHING**
  Appropriate, reserved, bright colours, self-neglect, exposing body excessively
- **CONVERSATION**
  Thought disorders, sexual content to delusions, sexually gratifying acts
- **PHYSICAL ILLNESS**
  - Neurological, endocrine, cardiac, respiratory, neoplasms
  - Psychotropic and physical medications may impair sexual function and cause euphoria, disinhibition and, especially in the elderly, delirium
- **MENTAL STATE**
  Elation, hallucinations, delusional beliefs, depression, anxiety, gratification from act, aggressive, sadistic personality traits
- **Approaching other patients or public asking for sexual activity**
- **Sexually explicit conversation**
- **Low intelligence level and cognitive impairment suggest impaired judgement**

DIFFERENTIAL DIAGNOSIS

Psychiatric

- Bipolar disorder: manic episode; depressive episode less common
- Schizophrenia: sexualized behaviour in response to hallucinations or delusions
- Delusional disorder
- Learning difficulties: impaired judgement
- Exhibitionism as an aggressive act; may precede sexual assault or as only means of sexual gratification

Organic

- Delirium
- Dementia (especially Pick's disease)
- Organic mood disorder: manic episode. Frontal lobe dysfunction (tumour, multiple sclerosis, medication)
- Psychoactive substance misuse (drug and alcohol, but stimulants more likely to cause this)

IMMEDIATE MANAGEMENT

- Sexual disinhibition may arise in the context of elation, when it is goal-directed behaviour, or in a disorganized state of delirium or dementia. It may also arise as a clumsy attempt to be intimate when there is impaired judgement because of either dementia or learning difficulties. These situations may arise in A & E, on a ward or in the community. In the latter case either a member of the public or the police are likely to become involved. The police are most likely to be involved if an offence is committed: exhibitionism, sexual assaults, including rape. Those individuals who are clearly suffering from a mood disorder or impaired judgement in the absence of any offence are likely to be guided to hospitals for treatment without charges being pressed
- The immediate management involves ensuring the safety of the individual and the public. The individual may not be in touch with reality. Obtain as detailed a history as possible, taking account of how the elation and a grandiose mental state may affect the information given. Medical, psychiatric and drug history are essential. Informants should be interviewed at every opportunity to establish the time course of the behaviours causing concern. A chronic course suggests dementia. A sudden onset should alert the clinician to the possibility of a physical illness or drug intoxication. Specific details about mood, content of hallucinations and delusional thinking will be important if charges are pressed for any reason. For serious offences, discuss the case with forensic services. A cognitive assessment is essential; if there is any evidence of significantly impaired intelligence, specialist learning difficulty services should be involved. If there is evidence of delirium, this should be treated as a medical emergency. A full physical examination (especially neurological) should be performed. The patient may be in a state of acute distress if assaulted. Admission for treatment of mood disorder or investigation is likely to be necessary

THE SUBSTANCE-MISUSING PATIENT

Patients may present themselves to A & E departments, their GP practice or their families. Alternatively they may be brought to the attention of a psychiatric team by probation officers, social services or the police because of violent behaviour, criminal offences, suicide attempts or obvious distress in public. Patients are often temporary residents and seek drugs out of hours.

SYMPTOMS AND CLINICAL SIGNS

- **PATTERN OF INTERACTION WITH DRUG**
  - Intoxication or withdrawal
  - Conscious feigning of symptoms to obtain substances with or without self-medication
- **SPECIFIC PSYCHOBEHAVIOURAL SIGNS AND SYMPTOMS**
  - **Heightened sense of well-being**: impulsive, reckless and unpredictable behaviour
  - **Violence**: as a consequence of a paranoid psychosis or personality disorder and demands refused. Agitation and overactivity are predisposing factors
  - **Delirium**: acute intoxication with any drug but exclude Ecstasy and cocaine, which can be fatal; withdrawal symptoms can also present thus
  - **Psychiatric symptoms** may be caused by substances but dual diagnoses should be considered: hallucinations, paranoia, anxiety states, depressive symptoms with or without attempts at suicide and deliberate self-harm
  - **Personality disorders**: convictions and forensic history; repeated acts of violence against people or property with no evidence of mental disorder
- **PHYSICAL SIGNS AND SYMPTOMS**
  - Changes in consciousness level, fever, tachycardia, hypertensive and hypotensive states, cardiac murmurs, needle marks, lymphadenopathy, abscess, pupils dilated or constricted, constipation, diarrhoea
  - **Complications**: pneumonia, HIV-positive, persistent generalized lymphadenopathy (PGL) and AIDS, hepatitis-B- or -C-positive, fits, respiratory arrest, accidental overdose, septicaemia, infective endocarditis, osteomyelitis, thrombophlebitis, viral infections, dermatological complaints including skin abscess, allergic reactions

DIFFERENTIAL DIAGNOSIS

Dual diagnoses are common.

Psychiatric

- Paranoid schizophrenia
- Bipolar affective disorder: manic episode
- Personality disorder: dissocial
- Munchausen syndrome/malingering: may be related to criminality

Organic

- **Delirium**: head injury, epileptic automatism, HIV-related dementia, acute confusion
- **Drug intoxication**: opiate, cocaine, Ecstasy, LSD, amphetamines, cannabis, solvents, alcohol

IMMEDIATE MANAGEMENT

- The priority is to exclude coexistent physical illness. If present this needs to be treated alongside any psychiatric symptoms. Problems of acute intoxication and withdrawal include delirium, psychosis, violence. Treatment of withdrawal states may alleviate aggression, anxiety, confusion and psychosis. If there are accompanying behavioural problems or risk to the patient or others because of aggression with or without psychotic symptoms, then an admission should be arranged
- Liaison with specialist drug agencies at the earliest opportunity is essential for the setting of realistic admission objectives and implementation of aftercare plans
- A contract regarding the availability of all drugs (prescribed and non-prescribed) should be carefully constructed as part of the agreed admission aims. In the absence of an urgent admission, each department should have a specific policy regarding the prescribing of drugs of misuse to addicts. **Avoid prescribing unless there are clear signs of withdrawal.** Outpatient referral to a specialist team should be made and the GP should be informed as soon as possible of the contact and of any prescribed drugs. Non-opiates may be successfully used for the symptomatic treatment of opiate withdrawal (propranolol, Lomotil, thioridazine, paracetamol). If already on a reducing regimen and there are clear signs of withdrawal, and the decision to prescribe methadone has been taken, then the elixir is preferred. Prescribe only sufficient to avoid a crisis, with early involvement of a single agency and keyworker (from primary care or specialist services) to coordinate the total aftercare package. If there are no signs of withdrawal, do not prescribe methadone as an emergency
- If consciousness level is impaired through intoxication, an admission for observation is necessary to exclude dehydration, respiratory and cardiovascular collapse, especially if cocktails (e.g. opiates, solvents or 'crack' cocaine) have been used
- **Deliberate self-harm and suicide**: assess suicidal risk. Admission under the Mental Health Act may be necessary if suicidality is due to mental illness
- **Pregnancy**: antenatal care may not have been taken up. This opportunity could be used to engage with obstetric services. If withdrawal symptoms are present, there is a risk of premature labour and an admission for assessment by paediatrician, obstetrician and specialist drug services should be arranged

REFERENCES

1. Morgan HG, Priest P. Assessment of suicide risk in psychiatric inpatients. Br J Psychiatry 1984; 145: 467–469. Although about inpatients, remains essential reading.
2. Pierce D. Suicidal intent and repeated self harm. Psychol Med 1984; 14: 655–659.

SECTION III

Psychiatric Wards and Accident and Emergency Departments

ACCIDENT AND EMERGENCY DEPARTMENTS

SECTORIZATION

Geographically defined areas (sectors) have been identified and implemented as the core unit around which psychiatric services are planned and delivered. Each sector has a single team of health-care professionals. This not only facilitates an accurate evaluation of service shortfalls but also attempts to deliver care to patients within the locality of their own communities. A single named team, named keyworker and named consultant then become responsible for a patient throughout their residence within any one geographical area. This ensures continuity of care for the severely mentally ill requiring longer-term rehabilitative care focused on their own unique profile of disabilities. In some localities sector boundaries coincide with social services' boundaries so that care can be more effectively and jointly planned and delivered. Where this arrangement does not exist, greater difficulties are encountered when coordinating a comprehensive package of care.[1]

HOMELESSNESS

Between 30% and 50% of the homeless population has been identified as suffering from significant mental illness.[2] Such patients may have a history of unstable accommodation because they are unable to coordinate their own affairs or their symptoms are not acceptable to landlords and neighbours and no one attempts to find them accommodation at the appropriate level of support. Because of their intransigence or challenging behaviour, such patients may not have a GP. These patients have multiple needs but in view of their geographical instability they are likely to see many doctors and teams without one team remaining in charge of their care regardless of address. Mental health teams concerned with the homeless are being established to address the physical and psychiatric care needs of this population. Such teams should be involved, especially on admission, as they may be able to offer continuity of care. Hostels also have specific GPs who attend to the physical care of certain patients. Once admitted to hospital, accommodation with appropriate level of support should be pursued and this task should begin on admission by a referral to the sector social-work team for a needs assessment. There may also be other social and physical problems. On discharge all problem areas should be addressed in the discharge plan as in this group failure to meet any one need may compromise all other interventions. When assessing homeless patients, enquire in detail about accommodation type, quality, size, length of residence, tenancy. Focus on inadequacies of the accommodation and question whether remedying these shortfalls would avoid or reduce the length of admission. Seek as much information as possible from all sources, such as hostel workers, GP, friends, neighbours and informal carers.

ESTABLISHING RESIDENCE

For those with stable addresses and not under the care of any mental-health team, their current address should be looked up in the local (hospital-based) directory of catchment areas. Such a directory should be available on each ward and in A & E, and a copy should be available for each duty doctor. A single responsible medical officer (RMO – the consultant) is responsible for each sector. When patients are homeless their most recent address serves as the working address for health and social-care arrangements. Where patients are already under the care of a mental health team they remain the team's responsibility until a formal transfer of responsibility has taken place (team to team and RMO to RMO). Establishing residence is vital as soon as contact is made as this determines which agencies and professionals are likely to be involved. If the patient is brought to A & E by the police because of an offence, the site of offence can serve as the point of residence. This also applies to convicted homeless patients who are awaiting diversion to psychiatric hospitals.

MODELS OF WORKING WITH ACCIDENT AND EMERGENCY STAFF

'Walk-in' clinic

- Psychiatrist sees all who seek a psychiatric opinion. No screening
- Senior psychiatric nurse screens all who wish to see a psychiatric professional and refers only those needing to see a psychiatrist
- Psychiatrist sees all but deals with psychiatric needs only and refers physical care to casualty officer
- Psychiatrist sees all referrals and deals with physical and psychiatric problems

Standard accident and emergency

- Screened by casualty triage staff and referred direct to psychiatrist
- Screened by casualty staff, referred to casualty officer who refers to psychiatrist
- Managed by casualty officer and referred only if casualty officer wants a specialist opinion

GP referrals come in by either route and may follow direct referral to psychiatrist, casualty officer or with no direct referral. The latter is likely if there is known to be a 'walk-in' clinic.

Establish clearly what the local procedures are. This avoids endless surprises and frustration with colleagues who may be acting within locally agreed procedural guidelines not known to you. If the procedures are not working because of workload, inappropriate referrals or because the needs of certain groups of patients cannot be met within the local model, then instigate change by discussion with senior staff in the A & E and psychiatric departments. It may be time to review the guidelines.

SOURCES OF INFORMATION

Exploit all sources of accessible information to evaluate the accuracy of the history given, previous interventions that have succeeded or failed before constructing a treatment plan. Contact previous wards, to access previous notes. Some staff members who know your patient well may be on the wards. Old notes should be obtained wherever possible and certainly should be requested if at another hospital. Contact the patient's last consultant and keyworker. If in supported accommodation discuss the options with the housing staff, who otherwise may be left to deal with an unworkable treatment plan. If there are social needs, identify the allocated social worker or probation services if a forensic history emerges. Always speak with the GP and relatives. They may have the most complete information and be able to list previous interventions and coping strategies for persistent symptoms. Any treatment plan must take account of the relatives' and GP's involvement.

INTERVIEWING AND SAFETY

Violent assault is not uncommon in psychiatric settings, medical settings and other public services. In one study, 41% of junior doctors had experienced physical violence and 36% had suffered physical injuries; 63% had experienced verbal violence.[3] Ensure that the interview room you are about to use is in sight of other staff, and has an alarm button that works and is accessible. Tell other staff you are about to use the interview room. If you anticipate problems, do not interview by yourself, however pressed for time you or other staff may be. Ask another staff member to join you. Preferably, this should be a psychiatric nurse but in some instances security guards are the only people available. If in doubt, interview in an open place while making an initial assessment of dangerousness. Never rush into closed interview rooms with people who may be acutely disturbed or whom you suspect of potential malice. If you are frightened then you cannot carry out a sensible assessment, so defer until someone can accompany you.

TRAINING AND SAFETY

Most organizations should hold training workshops on how to deal with potentially violent members of the public, who may or may not be patients. This should include strategies such as talking down, taking up non-threatening body postures, reminding the potential assailant of your ordinary human qualities, such as your name, considering escape techniques and survival strategies should you be taken hostage, raising the alarm, and sources of support and information about counselling after such a crisis. The use of personal alarms is advisable for men and women; do not walk around isolated hospital sites on your own at night. Ask for an escort from security. Bravado will blind you to the potential dangers. The same advice can be applied to home visits. Do not try to disarm anyone yourself. Ask the individual to give up any weapons and tell them that you are unable to see them until all weapons have been handed in. Ask the police to assist.

WORKING ON PSYCHIATRIC WARDS

ATTEMPTED SUICIDE

The Department of Health's *The Health of the Nation* targets for suicide prevention were:

- to reduce the overall rate by 15% by the year 2000
- in the severely mentally ill, to reduce the rate by 33% by the year 2000.

Half the people who kill themselves have a current or past psychiatric illness. 'Not all suicides can be prevented, even within the best-run psychiatric wards'.[4] Inpatients at risk should not be discharged prematurely because of symptomatic improvement alone, as this may be misleading and may be followed by relapse on discharge. Alienation of patients can hinder delivery of appropriate levels of care and supervision. In these instances, setting boundaries and handing back responsibility to the patient, although a valuable and effective skill when judiciously applied, may be counter-therapeutic. Admission is necessary for those for whom other community-based interventions have failed and/or the risk of completed suicide is too high to justify community management. Changes in the level of supervision, unresolved psychosocial conflicts and non-compliance with medication and failure of follow-up are other factors of relevance in completed suicide after discharge. There are few single services that can deliver all the components of what is regarded as an optimal package of interventions.

SUICIDE RATES

The annual rates have been increasing in the UK: 48 per 100 000 in 1920/21 to 84 per 100 000 in 1972/73. Although the rates for women have decreased recently, the rates among specific groups, e.g. young Asian women and young black men, have been increasing steadily. While on the ward, 1.3–2.5 patients per 1000 discharges complete suicide.[5] The relative risks of suicide are elevated for young men with schizophrenia (49 times), women with affective psychoses (91 times) and men and women with neuroses (33 times).[6] Social factors such as unemployment, isolation, recent bereavement or separation, being male, elderly or living alone add to the risk, irrespective of mental illness. Alcoholism and drug misuse account for up to 29% of inpatient suicides.

Patients will use methods that are readily available and adapt anything in the ward environment: overdoses of concealed tablets, drowning in baths, hanging, self-cutting, jumping off high buildings and out of windows. Setting fires, although less common, is a possibility; if there is a history of fire-setting ensure materials to start a fire are removed. On admission ensure that all potential weapons (razor blades, belts, etc.) are given up.

PRECAUTIONS AND OBSERVATION POLICY

The ward environment should be carefully planned so as to avoid the high-risk and observation rooms being placed near to opening windows and staircases. Good observational access is essential without being too intrusive. A calm ward atmosphere is necessary, as admission on to an acutely disturbed ward will not enable a distressed patient to settle and indeed will distract staff from providing optimal care to each patient. Well-kept, decorated open spaces, low, comfortable seats and well-lit wards will encourage patients to stay voluntarily and enable them to feel contained and safe.

On admission, assess suicide risk carefully, and make explicit your concerns to the patient, relatives and staff. Ensure that the level of support and supervision during the early stage of admission takes account of the risk factors (and that the keyworker has not yet established a rapport with the patient). Document the level of observation and communicate it verbally to the keyworker. Each unit has specific observation policies. Ensure that both you and the keyworker have the same understanding of the terms 'special observation' and 'continuous observation'. Set the frequency of visual and interpersonal vigilance as well as the time of commencement, and review these levels of observation in the light of nursing reports. Anticipate reasons why the level of observation might need to be increased or decreased earlier. Clearly state which changes to the treatment plan can be sanctioned without you reassessing the patient. Set a time at which the plan, including an assessment of risk, will be reviewed in the light of the immediately preceding assessment period.

At a managerial level there should be adequate staffing numbers to ensure that adequate supervision and support can be delivered. If there is a completed suicide, alert senior staff immediately; do not alter old notes, and immediately make a fresh entry outlining in as much detail as possible the circumstances of the incident and the impressions that the clinical staff had developed regarding the risk of suicide when the patient was last seen. Arrange a full multidisciplinary meeting away from the ward to critically analyse the incident for audit purposes. Examine supportively what procedures and mechanisms were unsuccessful and which additional measures are necessary.

REPEATED SELF-CUTTING

This can reach epidemic proportions within hospital units. Such self-harm can take the form of superficial cutting with little suicidal intent; deeper cuts that endanger major vessels are not always linked to serious intent; bizarre unpredictable acts of self-mutilation are more common among psychotic people and may be fatal if deep cuts are made near to major vessels. Self-cutters tend to be young, female, to come from broken homes and to have relationship difficulties, may have been subjected to physical and sexual abuse, have few close trusting relationships, may have been subject to early childhood illness, and may have contact with the paramedical professions.

People may cut:

- impulsively in order to end an intolerable experience
- because of severe anxiety, anger or agitation
- for a sense of relief that accompanies the cutting and the sight of blood (perhaps mediated by endogenous release of opiates and adrenaline) and

- where there are distortions of thinking that are depressive in nature and that morbidly rationalize the cutting as the first step in recovery or as a punishment that must be accepted.

Ensure that the necessary emergency assessment and treatment of lacerations is carried out before considering the psychiatric management. A behavioural analysis of the sequence of cutting is essential to identify precipitants as well as protective factors. Assess impulsivity, ability to verbalize and explore feelings, distorted cognitions and rationalization, depth of cuts, target areas cut, associated suicidal intent and risk of accidental suicide in the absence of active intent. Make yourself aware of all past acts, motives, social stressors, comorbid states (moods, alcohol misuse), behavioural precursors and coping strategies. Interventions include cognitive therapies, communication work, physical exercise, relaxation techniques, allaying of social stressors and treating depressogenic cognitions as well as other depressive symptoms. Medications include antidepressants, neuroleptics, lithium and carbamazepine. A behavioural contract should be drawn up to effectively link all the strategies.

MANAGEMENT ROUNDS

Models of management rounds

Multidisciplinary management (or ward) rounds have been a common component in the assessment and treatment of psychiatric inpatients. Such rounds include the medical team (consultant, senior registrar, registrar, senior house officer, medical students), nursing staff (primary nurse of each patient along with a senior member of nursing staff, nursing students), social workers (a single one attached to the team or several who visit when their particular patients are being discussed), occupational therapists, psychologists, pharmacists and liaising members of other medical, nursing or social care teams. In the UK the junior doctor traditionally has had the responsibility of making available all the necessary information to facilitate problem-based decision-making. This approach is modelled on the role of a junior doctor in the medical profession in the UK generally. Other disciplines either present their own findings or feed back to the junior doctor or another team member. In specialist units only one or two patients may be presented in each round and discussed in great detail but in standard psychiatric units usually all patients are discussed, with special attention given to newly admitted patients. Patients may or may not all be seen during the round. Such a process has always been put forward as an efficient way of collating all necessary opinions and making joint interagency decisions on a once-a-week basis. Although this approach has been the mainstay of inpatient psychiatry in the UK for many years, the majority of patients prefer not to attend or to have an alternative style of round.[7] Also, the extent of nurse involvement is sometimes deemed to be insufficient; professional hierarchies are often blamed for limiting the effectiveness of the rounds.[8] The use of management rounds for teaching purposes has also been questioned.[9]

Many clinicians now choose to meet with patients separately, as do other members of the team, so that the round becomes a decision-making one establishing the framework for care, with the primary nurse acting as the patient's advocate. The outcome of the meeting is then discussed with the patient separately and agreed plans are then initiated.

Functions of management rounds

The functions of management rounds include: decision-making about medication and psychological therapies; discussion about indications for specific interventions and the impact of any interventions; integration of all the information so far available about the patient's social, psychological and physical well-being; team building, making links with other teams to make or receive face-to-face referrals; and case conferences. Teaching students and mutual exchange of information are other less noticed functions. Meeting and explaining the treatment rationale to family members is another less commonly cited function. Shorter problem-solving management rounds involving the core inpatient treatment team are increasingly common, lending support to the view that treatment decisions should be made more often if a patient's progress is not to be impeded because of the administrative structure of a unit. Daily problem-solving rounds involving junior and some senior staff are becoming increasingly popular in view of the pressure to vacate inpatient beds, the greater complexity of patient problems presented and the level of disturbance on wards, all reflecting the need to review treatment plans more often in order to optimize progress.

Clinical tasks of the junior doctor

- Collate all the necessary information from the admission and progress notes and investigations
- Do the admission assessments
- Liaise with other medical and nursing staff if physical care is necessary
- Liaise effectively with other ward staff (all disciplines) so as to ensure that patients receive the appropriate level of care from other disciplines
- Plan discharge arrangements in conjunction with all parties likely to be involved in delivering future care
- Communicate effectively with GPs
- Prepare summaries (admission and discharge)
- Provide emergency and routine physical care
- Record the process and content of the management round and section 117 meetings

Treatment plans and section 117 meetings

Section 117 of the Mental Health Act 1983 requires that social services, healthcare services and all voluntary organizations involved in care should agree procedures for establishing aftercare arrangements.[10] The keyworker coordinates the time and venue of the meeting. Participants include the RMO (consultant), the primary nurse who looks after the patient while in hospital, a social worker specializing in mental health work, the GP, the community psychiatric nurse, who will be coordinating the community care package, a member of any relevant voluntary organization and the patient and/or a member of their family or an advocate. Each hospital should have agreed procedures for carrying out these meetings and recording the process and outcome. Such planning meetings are essential for those patients who are potentially violent, have forensic histories, have been admitted on a Mental Health Act section or are vulnerable in view of their continuing mental health and social care needs.[11]

MULTIDISCIPLINARY TEAMS

The emergence of diverse models of mental illness and the development of comprehensive treatment packages highlighted the fact that the care of psychiatric patients could only be optimized if the expertise from a number of professional disciplines is harnessed and effectively applied to supply the best possible care. Community mental health teams have been deemed to be the best way of providing for the specialist needs of certain client groups and also the best way to improve cooperation and collaboration between professionals and agencies.

TYPES OF TEAM[12–14]

- Those that deliver direct care shaped by the needs of clients
- Those that develop and support other services necessary for clients (e.g. preventative or early intervention services)
- Combinations of the above two approaches depending upon the degree to which respective management and professional structures allow teams to function independently
- Teams may also be funded largely from one body or have an excess of one profession; the functional success will then be influenced by the dominant group's ideology

Good team organization requires that there be an operational policy including 'targeted' groups and a mission statement, a definition of the geographical sector and the component team functions, team procedures for receiving and making referrals and discharging clients. Team membership, accountability and supervision structures must be explicit. Team meetings need an agreed structure and decision-making process. Team members' roles need to be specified. Team administration procedures need to be agreed. Individual carer and team development should be accommodated and attention given to 'burnout' and 'stress management' among team members.

WHEN THINGS GO WRONG

Dual accountability and influences may lead to role conflict for an individual or for several members of a team. Unless the management of such conflict is anticipated, poor interpersonal relationships within a team could undermine effective functioning. Fragmentation and burnout are signs of failing team processes and should be identified and dealt with early with a view to the team agreeing to take positive and creative steps to overcome obstacles. Functions within a team may extend beyond or fall short of the roles that any one professional group would regard as acceptable for its profession. The effective management of risk, with dangerous patients for example, needs clear lines of accountability and responsibility, especially where a team usually has much greater flexibility of roles suited to better management of less risky patients. A greater emphasis on operational policies, where key agencies and professionals in a multidisciplinary team have their responsibilities and lines of accountability are specified, can prevent such breakdowns of team working.[13,14]

RELATIVES

Families are the main source of support for the majority of the mentally ill. To avoid burnout among family members, so that they can continue to be effective in their roles as carers, they need adequate and continuous support, information, timely respite and sufficient time from professionals for consultation. Relatives can provide a vast amount of information for any first presentation; family members have special knowledge of the culture from which an individual comes and they will have their own opinions about the cause of the illness and potential solutions. These should be elicited. The use of a non-blaming approach and developing a working alliance with families as well as the patient is essential.

Several studies have demonstrated lower relapse rates where family interventions are combined with neuroleptic treatment. The concept of high expressed emotion as measured by the Camberwell Family Assessment Interview has been the focus of attention as a very valuable intervention. Other approaches to family working that do not give so much attention to expressed emotion have been shown to be effective and less likely to be misunderstood as blaming the family. Yet both approaches appear to be hampered in practice by the availability of staff with specialist training in these areas.

Involve family members in medication-related decisions – the reasons for prescribing and the adverse and therapeutic effects of medication, but also the limitations of it. Family education, communication and problem solving seem to be important ingredients when combined with case management and work with the individual. This approach is especially important where treatment decisions are controversial, where the illness appears to be resistant to standard treatment approaches or where special circumstances make direct communication with the patient difficult (e.g. hard of hearing, thought-disordered patients, ethnic minorities, uncommunicative patients).

REFERENCES

1. Thornicroft G. The case for catchment areas for mental health services. Psychiatr Bull 1995; 19: 343–345.
2. Scott J. Homeless and mental illness. Br J Psychiatry 1993; 162: 314–324.
3. Schneiden V. Violence against doctors. Br J Hosp Med 1993; 50: 6–9.
4. Morgan HG. Suicide prevention. Hazards on the fast lane to community care. Br J Psychiatry 1992; 160: 149–153.
5. Morgan G. Suicide in psychiatric hospitals. In: Hawton K, Cowen P, eds. Dilemmas and difficulties in the management of psychiatric patients. Oxford: Oxford University Press, 1990.
6. King E. Suicide in the mentally ill. Br J Psychiatry 1994; 165: 658–663.
7. Foster HD, Falkowski W, Rollings J. A survey of patient attitudes towards inpatient psychiatric ward rounds. Int J Social Psychiatry 1991; 37: 135–140.
8. Busby A, Gilchrist B. The role of the nurse in the medical ward round. J Adv Nurs 1992; 17: 339–346.
9. Elliot D, Hickam D. Attending rounds on in-patient units: differences between medical and non-medical services. Med Educ 1993; 27: 503–508.
10. Department of Health and Welsh Office. Code of Practice. Mental Health Act 1983. London: HMSO, 1990.
11. Royal College of Psychiatrists. Good medical practice in the aftercare of potentially violent or vulnerable patients discharged from inpatient psychiatric treatment. London: Royal College of Psychiatrists, 1991.
12. Ovretveit J. Making the team work. Prof Nurse 1994; 5(6): 284–288.
13. Ovretveit J, Temple H, Coleman R. The organization and management of community mental health teams. London: Good Practices in Mental Health, 380–384 Harrow Road, and Guildford; Interdisciplinary Association of Mental Health Workers, Department of Educational Studies, University of Surrey.
14. Onyett S. Responsibility and accountability in community mental health teams. Psychiatr Bull 1995; 19: 281–285.

SECTION IV

The Mental Health Act

Table 2 *Civil sections*

Section	Title	Duration	Grounds	Recommendation	Application	Discharge
2	Admission for assessment or assessment followed by treatment	Up to 28 days from admission	Mental disorder of nature or degree that warrants detention in hospital for a limited period and detained in interests of own health or safety or that of others	Two doctors, one section-12-approved, within 5 days of each other. Admit within 14 days of last recommendation. One doctor should have previous knowledge of patient. Second doctor must not be from same hospital	Nearest relative ASW (within 14 days of date of application	RMO Hospital managers Nearest relative giving 72 hours notice but if doctors deem such action to be dangerous this can be barred pending a manager's hearing MHRT: Nearest relative within 28 days Patient within 14 days of detention
3	Admission for treatment	Up to 6 months, renewable after 6 months and then annually	Mental illness, mental impairment, severe mental impairment or psychopathic disorder Of nature or degree that makes it appropriate for him or her to receive medical treatment in hospital Necessary for health or safety of patient and/or protection of others And for PD and mental impairment – treatment likely to alleviate or prevent deterioration	As for section 2 One doctor must be approved under section 12(2)	As for section 2 If nearest relative objects, ASW cannot make application but if objection is unreasonable then the ASW may apply to county court to remove the nearest relative	As for section 2 MHRT: Nearest relative within 28 days of RMO barring their right to discharge By patient within 6 months Hospital managers will refer for appeal after 6 months anyway if no previous appeal

Table 2 *Civil sections (continued)*

Section	Title	Duration	Grounds	Recommendation	Application	Discharge
4	Admission in emergency for assessment	Up to 72 hours from admission on the understanding that section 2 will be organized on admission	As in section 2 plus urgent necessity	Nearest relative or ASW, one doctor, preferably with previous knowledge, within 24 hours of seeing patient	Nearest relative or ASW seen within last 24 hours	After 72 hours, unless second medical recommendation that complies with requirements of section 2
5(4)	Nurse holding power	6 hours from record of decision in writing	Appears to be suffering from mental disorder to such a degree that for their health or safety, or that of others, should be immediately restrained from leaving hospital and not practicable to get section 5(2)	Nurse of prescribed class (RMN in charge of ward)		Ceases on arrival of section 3 doctor. Patient may leave or be discharged unless further detained
5(2)	Detention of patient already in hospital	72 hours (including start of nurse holding power)		Doctor in charge of the case, or his/her nominated deputy (therefore, does not have to be a psychiatrist)		Must be discharged within 72 hours unless further powers of detention are enacted

ASW, approved social worker; MHRT, Mental Health Act Review Tribunal; PD, psychopathic disorder; RMN, registered mental nurse; RMO, responsible medical officer.

***Table 3** Forensic sections*

Section	Title	Diagnostic groups	Grounds	Application	Duration
35	Remand to hospital for a report on the accused's mental condition	Mental illness, psychopathic disorder, mental impairment or severe mental impairment	*Crown Courts* If awaiting trial for an offence punishable by imprisonment (other than murder) *Magistrates' court* If convicted of an offence punishable on summary conviction with imprisonment If charged with such an offence (if the court is satisfied that he or she committed the act or made the omission or if he or she has consented to the exercise of the power) If court is satisfied that it would be impracticable to obtain such a report while on bail The patient must be admitted within 7 days of the date of remand	Criminal Courts: One medical practitioner approved under section 12(2)	Up to 28 days. Renewable in 28-day periods up to a maximum of 12 weeks. This is not a treatment order and a person remanded cannot be treated without his or her consent
36	Remand of an accused person to hospital for treatment	Mental illness or severe mental impairment only	*Crown Courts* As above for section 35 Mental illness or severe mental impairment of a nature or degree which makes it appropriate for him or her to be detained in hospital for medical treatment The patient will be admitted within 7 days of the date of remand	Crown Courts only: Two medical practitioners; one must be approved under section 12(2)	As section 35, but can be treated without his or her consent in accordance with Part IV

Table 3 *Forensic sections (continued)*

Section	Title	Diagnostic groups	Grounds	Application	Duration
37	Powers of the courts to order hospital admission or guardianship	As for section 35	*Crown Courts* Any person convicted and punishable by imprisonment (other than murder) *Magistrates' court* If convicted of an offence punishable on summary conviction with imprisonment If charged with such an offence (if the court is satisfied that he or she committed the act or made the omission or if he or she has consented to the exercise of the power) If the offender's mental disorder is of a nature or degree which makes it appropriate for him or her to be detained in hospital for medical treatment In the case of psychopathy or mental impairment, if such treatment is likely to alleviate or prevent deterioration in his or her condition If the patient will be admitted within 28 days of the order, and the Region can be expected to specify when the bed will be available	Criminal Courts: As for section 36, but the court must be satisfied on the written or oral evidence of the RMO or the hospital managers that the admission criteria are satisfied	As for section 3: 6 months; can be extended by the RMO by 6 months and thereafter for a year at a time. All patients admitted under a hospital order may appeal to the Crown or Appeal Court. The patient can be discharged by the RMO, hospital managers or MHRT
38	Interim hospital order to assess suitability of making a hospital order	As for section 35	As for section 37 but magistrates' court cannot make such an order on unconvicted persons And that there is reason to suppose that the mental disorder is such that it may be appropriate to make a hospital order	Criminal Courts: As for section 36 but one medical practitioner must be employed by the admitting hospital	Initially up to 12 weeks, followed by periods of 28 days up to a maximum of 6 months. May be converted into a section 37 hospital order by the courts at any stage

Table 3 Forensic sections (continued)

Section	Title	Diagnostic groups	Grounds	Application	Duration
41	Order by higher courts to restrict movements after discharge from hospital (with or without limit of time)	As for section 35	Only for hospital orders The court has to consider the nature of the offence, the antecedents of the offender, the risk of committing further offences if discharged, and the protection of the public from serious harm	Crown Courts only: As for section 36, but one medical practitioner must give oral evidence to the court	Discharge by RMO or managers only with consent of the Home Secretary. Discharged by Home Secretary or MHRT. RMO must furnish the Home Office with an annual report on the patient
47	Transfer sentenced prisoners to hospital	As for section 35. Home Secretary must be satisfied that transfer of prisoner is expedient considering public interest	As for the criteria for section 37: That the offender's mental disorder is of a nature or degree that makes it appropriate for him or her to be detained in hospital for medical treatment In the case of psychopathy or mental impairment, if such a treatment is likely to alleviate or prevent deterioration in his or her condition The prisoner must be admitted within 14 days of the order	Home Secretary As for section 36	As for section 37
48	Transfer remand prisoners to hospital	As for section 36	As for additional criterion for section 37: That the offender's mental disorder is of a nature or degree that makes it appropriate for him to be detained in hospital for medical treatment The prisoner must be in need of urgent treatment	Home Secretary As for section 36	Until either the accused's case has been dealt with by the court or he or she has been returned to prison because of recovery from mental disorder
49	Transfer from prison to hospital with restrictions on discharge	As for section 35	As for section 41 but applied to a section 47	Home Secretary As for section 36	The patient can be returned to prison if Home Secretary requests it. The restriction order ceases to have effect at what would have been the earliest release date, when the section 47/49 becomes in effect a section 37 hospital order

MHRT, Mental Health Act Review Tribunal; RMO, responsible medical officer.

CIVIL AND FORENSIC SECTIONS

These sections of the Act are detailed in the tables on pp. 58–59 and 60–62.

CONSENT TO TREATMENT RULES

The Mental Health Act specifies that medical treatments include care, rehabilitation under medical supervision, physical treatments such as medication and ECT, and psychotherapy. Before any treatment can be given, valid consent of the patient must be obtained unless common law or statute law sanctions lawful treatment without consent. For those on a detention order (section 2 or 3 or 37) treatment can be given, for mental disorder only, without consent for the first 3 months of the order. At 3 months the RMO must complete a form 38 (certifying that the patient consents) or seek the completion of form 39 (if the patient refuses treatment), when a second opinion must be sought from the Mental Health Act Commission. Treatment for any physical illness falls outside the remit of the Mental Health Act and must be treated under common law. Blood samples that are necessary to ensure safety when treatment is given under a section of the Act are not covered by the Act but the commission has given guidelines that such precautions (taking blood samples) should be carried out to ensure safety until such time as a judicial review into the matter is held.

ELECTROCONVULSIVE THERAPY

Where the 3-month period has elapsed from the start of the section and treatment (usually medication) is still necessary, or where ECT is considered necessary under any circumstances (on or off section), and the patient does not consent or cannot give informed consent, the second opinion of a Mental Health Act Commissioner (MHAC) is necessary under section 58 of the Act. Only when the MHAC has completed a form 39 can treatment go ahead. In emergencies under section 62 of the Act urgent treatment that is not irreversible or hazardous may be given to save life or to prevent a severe deterioration or to prevent patients behaving violently or being a danger to themselves. Such treatment should be given once and once only in order to be the minimal interference necessary to save life. However, the Commission in practice accepts that, should the urgent situation arise again and a second opinion has not yet been secured then treatment under section 62 may be given on more than one occasion. However, as soon as a crisis is over, ordinary consent to treatment rules apply and a fresh application is necessary for each treatment.

PSYCHOSURGERY AND IMPLANTATION OF SEX HORMONES

These treatments cannot be given unless informed consent is given by the patient *and* an MHAC sanctions that the consent is valid (form 37 part 1) and that treatment is necessary (form 37 part 2). Such treatments are covered under section 57 of the Act. If a patient withholds or withdraws consent at any time, treatment cannot be given.

PLAN OF TREATMENT

Under section 59 of the Act, any treatment plan must be specified in whole or part in the patient's case notes and an outline will be included on the certificate. The MHAC may reject all or part of the plan. If the treatment plan is changed and the patient consents then a form 38 needs to be recompleted. If the patient does not consent then an MHAC's opinion and completion of form 39 is necessary to sanction the change in treatment.

THE MENTAL HEALTH ACT COMMISSIONER

When visiting to give a second opinion, the MHAC will need to meet with a nurse, a doctor, and one other professional concerned with the patient's care. He/she will also need to see the section papers, with any consent papers, and a clear treatment plan (signed by the RMO). A blank form 39 must be available for the commissioner. Having all of this in place will save much time and ensure that the visiting commissioner is fully informed of all the relevant information necessary to come to a decision.

CAPACITY TO GIVE CONSENT

In order to have 'capacity' a person must understand what the medical treatment is and why it is proposed in their instance. They should understand in general terms the nature of the treatment, its benefits and risks and the risks of not having the treatment. They should be able to exercise choice. 'Capacity' may vary over time and may vary if a person's mental state content interferes with their judgement about the intended treatment and their decision-making ability. The degree of capacity ascribed to an individual is essentially a clinical judgement informed by professional ethics, existing clinical practice and legislation. The definition is likely to change as professional practice, ethics and legal requirements are modified in light of advances in treatment and investigation and in light of specific rulings in instances where all these professional arenas fail to support a clear course of action and it is deemed necessary.

The 'capacity' required to make a decision must reflect the severity of the adverse outcomes if the wrong decision is made. So for a life-threatening illness maximum capacity is required. The presence of mental disorder does not alone indicate absence of capacity (although the Law Commission are considering this as one indicator) and it is clear that professionals are divided as to the best course of action in specific circumstances of potentially fatal medical illness and refusal of treatment in the absence of mental illness.[1] If in doubt, consult with a colleague, and make extensive notes about the content of the decision-making process, as well as any final decision. In cases of doubt an application to the High Court should be considered as one approach to secure a declaration that the proposed treatment is lawful.

ADVANCE STATEMENTS

The British Medical Association and the Royal Colleges have produced professional guidelines in the form of a code of practice and explanatory note about advance statements.[2] The code reflects the fact that advance statements are legally binding provided the person is competent to make such a statement, is not under duress and has contemplated potential later events, and that the statement does not require the doctor to act unlawfully. The implications for psychiatry include the early involvement of patients in the planning process when considering crisis management strategies, e.g. in anticipation of a deterioration in mental and physical health.

CHANGES IN THE LEGAL FRAMEWORK OF UK LAW

This section introduces the White Paper on new mental health legislation that was published in December 2000 in anticipation of a change to the Act; and introduces the relevant components of the Human Rights Act as it pertains to mental health practice. There were two recent changes that prompted calls for a review of mental health legislation:

- The bulk of care is now delivered in the community, with much effort by practitioners to not use inpatient hospital facilities
- The Human Rights Act, although signed up to some years ago by the British government, became enforceable in British courts in October 2000. Before then it was enforceable in European courts

These two significant changes prompted a call for a review of the Mental Health Act 1983, which was increasingly considered to be coercive and inappropriate for providing care in the community. There were also some reservations about its compatibility with the requirements of the Human Rights Act.

WHITE PAPER: *REFORMING THE MENTAL HEALTH ACT*

The White Paper, presented to Parliament in December 2000, emphasized changes in mental health legislation in the context of other changes in the National Health Service (NHS) and mental health services. Investment and service reform in line with the National Service Framework and the NHS Plan were seen to be necessary for changes in the Act to be meaningful.

Part 1: The new legal framework

Compulsory powers will be needed only if a person is resisting care and treatment is needed, either in their best interests or because without care and treatment they will pose a significant risk of serious harm to other people.

The legislation introduces:

- a new independent tribunal to determine all longer term compulsory powers
- a new right to independent advocacy
- new safeguards for people with long-term mental incapacity
- a new commission for mental health
- statutory requirements to develop care plans.

The new process is outlined in the box opposite. The new provisions allow care and treatment orders to apply to patients outside hospital. The intention is to prevent admission to hospital from being the only way to reinstate care plans. There will be no powers to give forcible treatment in a non-clinical setting (outside hospital) but steps will be taken to specify in community orders how patients will be prevented from becoming a risk to themselves, their carers or the public (if patients do not comply with the order). Some of the main features are as follows.

- Every patient must be informed of the powers that apply to them, and will have the right to free legal representation and advocacy (in the form of the new legal patient advocacy liaison service)
- There will also be a new duty of disclosure of information about patients suffering from mental disorder between health and social services and other agencies, including housing and criminal justice agencies
- In the care of children and adolescents, the new MHT will be obliged to seek specialist advice on health- and social-care aspects of the care plan. Decisions about children will take account of the general approach that a child's interests are paramount. There will be changes in the provisions for young persons aged between 16 and 18 in relation to refusal of consent to care and treatment of a mental disorder
- The clinical supervisor for a patient who might have long-term mental incapacity must carry out an assessment and obtain a second opinion

- A new commission for mental health will carry specific responsibilities for monitoring the use of formal powers, providing guidance on the operation of those powers and assuring the quality of training provided for practitioners with key responsibilities.

The new process leading to use of compulsory powers

- **STAGE 1: PRELIMINARY EXAMINATION**
  - By two doctors and a social worker (or other suitably trained mental health professional)
  - to consider if patient needs further assessment or urgent treatment by specialist mental health services
  - and that without this the patient might be at risk of serious harm or pose a risk of serious harm to other people
- **STAGE 2: FORMAL ASSESSMENT AND INITIAL TREATMENT UNDER COMPULSORY POWERS**
  - Full assessment in accord with a formal care plan
  - Initial period of assessment and treatment will be 28 days
  - After that any new detention must be authorised by a new independent decision-making body – the Mental Health Tribunal (MHT)
  - MHT obtains advice from independent experts and takes evidence from the clinical team, the patient and their representative, and other agencies
- **STAGE 3: CARE AND TREATMENT ORDER**
  - Tribunal or court will be able to make a care and treatment order, which will authorise the care and treatment specified in a care plan recommended by the clinical team
  - This must be designed:
    - to give a therapeutic benefit to the patient or
    - to manage behaviour associated with mental disorder that might lead to serious harm to other people

  The first two orders will be for 6 months and subsequent orders can be for 12 months

Part 2: High-risk patients

This part of the White Paper relates to the small numbers of people with mental disorder who pose a risk to others and are either detained under civil sections or remanded or convicted offenders. This includes people with personality disorders, who, by virtue of the treatability clause of the 1983 Act and the absence of specialist provision, were excluded from consideration under the powers of the current Act. The aims are to develop specialist services to address the needs of this client group, and to diminish risk to the public. The criteria for detention will distinguish between those who pose a risk to others and those where compulsory treatment is in their 'best interests'. Categories of mental disorder will not be defined so that, wherever there are concerns about mental disorder being sufficiently serious to warrant an assessment, without which there is risk to the public or risk to the patient's health, compulsory powers may be used. The care plan must be drawn up within 3 days of the decision to use compulsory powers.

The criteria will be that:

- The patient is diagnosed as having a mental disorder within the meaning of the new legislation
- The nature and degree of mental disorder warrants specialist care and treatment in the best interests of the patient and/or because without treatment there is significant risk of harm to others
- **Best interests of the patient**: the plan must be of direct therapeutic benefit to the patient
- **Risk to others**: the plan must be considered necessary either to directly treat the underlying mental disorder and/or to manage the behaviour arising from the disorder. Thus the care plan must include interventions that ameliorate the behaviours of concern, even when the underlying mental disorder can not be treated.

Controversy about the new Act

The need for a new Act is controversial: some psychiatrists consider that it extends coercive powers, which do not replace good practice, skills and properly resourced services. Furthermore, the new Act proposes special responsibilities to do with people who have personality disorder and pose a risk to the public. Hence, commentators are concerned that psychiatrists are being asked to 'police' social deviance in a way that community care was intended to end. Specifically, individuals can be detained to manage their behaviour in the absence of what might be considered a treatable mental illness, where dissocial personality disorder (DSPD) is considered a mental disorder. Specialist DSPD units may be set up to assist in assessment and treatment.

Discharge of high-risk patients must follow a risk assessment, with crisis plans that spell out the clinical supervisor's powers of recall to hospital should the community care plan not be followed. The new Criminal Justice and Court Services Act 2000 places a statutory duty on police and probation services to establish arrangements for assessing and managing the risks posed by sexual and violent dangerous offenders.

There will also be an obligation on primary care and community care trusts to assess individuals referred from probation, prisons, the police, carers and the courts.

The main concerns about legislative change are that it will work against engagement of those who are already over-represented in Mental Health Act detention statistics, and that it is clinical skills and collaborative relationships that are needed rather than new powers to detain and recall patients. Details of the Act will be specified in legislation and until then the 1983 Act is still in force.

THE HUMAN RIGHTS ACT 1998

This Act was signed over 50 years ago but was not part of British law until 1998 and only became enforceable in English courts in October 2000. The Act applies to all organizations and bodies but especially to public bodies. The Act presents a framework of principles by which life should be governed in countries that signed up to it. It is not prescriptive on details in law, but member countries must ensure that their laws and the operation of public bodies are consistent with the principles of the Act. Hence, there is no body of case law and this has to be developed by challenges to existing practice.

As far as mental health care is concerned, the Act mainly impacts on issues of self-determination and compulsory treatment. Prior to the Act consent to treatment rules were developed on the basis of case law and concluded that individuals refusing treatment must be able to comprehend and retain information, believe the information and weight it up to exercise choice. Rights to self-determination and liberty had to be balanced against the needs of the public and the right to receive treatment.

The Human Rights Act prohibits torture and inhumane or degrading treatment. It gives citizens a right to a fair trial, imposes a duty to respect family and private life, and suggests that interference is only justified under certain circumstances. The question arises as to whether psychiatric care is degrading or inhuman, and whether the failsafe mechanisms for those detained compulsorily are sufficiently robust. Criticism of tribunals and hospital environments have meant that each of these are also addressed in current health policy. The new Mental Health Act develops a substantial role for tribunals as independent bodies that will make legal decisions about long-term detention, rather than detention being determined only by clinical decisions previously made by professionals. Furthermore, article 5 says 'everyone has the right to liberty and security and ... no one shall be deprived of his liberty save in the following circumstances...'. Among these exceptions is the lawful detention of 'persons for the prevention of spreading of infectious diseases, ... persons of unsound mind, alcoholics and drug addicts or vagrants'. Thus the mentally ill, if considered to be of unsound mind, may be deprived of liberty, but such detention will be subject to legal challenges as afforded within the new Mental Health Act. A good summary of recent papers on both the Mental Health Act and the Human Rights Act can be found on http//:www//markwalton.net and the Department of Health website. The Sainsbury Centre for Mental Health has also produced a summary.

REFERENCES

1. Hardie T, Bhui K, Brown P. The emergency treatment of paracetamol overdose: a problem of consent to treatment. Psychiatr Bull 1995; 19: 7–9.
2. Feenan D. Advance statements about medical treatment. Br J Hosp Med 1995; 54: 107–109.

SECTION V

Liaison Psychiatry

THE WORK OF THE LIAISON PSYCHIATRIST

The daily reality of liaison for many juniors is the assessment of suicidal behaviour. Deliberate self-harm has been of central importance to the development of liaison psychiatry. It has been estimated that there are at least 100 000 hospital referrals per year in England and Wales for attempted suicide. The condition is the commonest reason for acute medical admission in females under 65 years and comes second only to ischaemic heart disease in men. Assessment of suicide risk is discussed on page 19.

Psychiatrists also have particular expertise in assessing challenging behaviours, including hostile, distressed and 'uncooperative' behaviour. As ever, the approach is to be systematic, succinct and respectful in one's opinion.

THE LIAISON ASSESSMENT

THE REFERRAL

- What for, why now, why worry? Why is this person being brought to my attention now? What are the major concerns about this person? What is the relevant history? Is there a history of challenging behaviours or self-harm? How does this person respond to new professionals or changes in his/her management?
- If it is not clear why you are being asked to see the patient, enquire politely of the referrer what they expect from your visit. The most frequent reasons for referral are:
  - Assessment of self-harm risk and mental state following overdose or other behaviour
  - Assessment of challenging behaviour – this includes hostility, anxiety, distress, withdrawal, refusal to cooperate with staff or treatment and perceived manipulative behaviour. All can usefully be considered within the rubric of abnormal illness behaviour
  - The patient has a pre-existing psychiatric illness for which management advice is required
  - The patient is thought to have a comorbid or secondary psychiatric disorder on which an opinion is being sought
  - There is diagnostic uncertainty
  - Somatization or conversion disorder is suspected
- Establish the urgency of the referral and how anxious staff are about the patient
- Establish whether the patient is expecting your visit – it is generally better if the patient has been primed. If necessary ask politely that the patient be told that a psychiatric opinion is being sought

- Examine the notes and talk to relevant staff to collect as much first-hand information as you can, particularly about:
  - Present diagnoses and treatment. What are the associations between this person's physical problems and management and psychiatric morbidity?
  - Past medical and psychiatric history
  - Premorbid personality and coping style
  - Role of developmental factors and life events
  - Somatization: does this person have medically unexplained physical symptoms? Is it appropriate to educate the patient to re-attribute their symptoms?
  - Attitudes of family/friends/carers/staff towards the episode
  - Social factors: what are the sources of external stress and support in this person's life? Consider particularly occupation, relationships, marital/cohabitation, family, social life, money, housing. What is the relevance of gender, ethnic and social class factors?
  - Organization of care: who currently sees this person, how often and what for? How often do they consult and what do they do?

THE INTERVIEW

- The interview skills are essentially as for any other psychiatric examination. Try to establish an appropriate level of privacy to interview the patient. See Section I for an approach to the mental state examination
- Structured interviews are widely available but opinions differ as to their merits (see p. 263)

THE REPORT

- Speak to the key nurse and referring doctor whenever possible and summarize your findings
- Write a succinct entry in the medical notes – essentially a formulation (see Section I on history-taking and note-keeping). Cover diagnoses, investigations, suggested physical, psychological and social management, if and when you will be seeing the patient again and who the relevant psychiatric contact point should be. More than one side of paper is probably too much. Further information can be conveyed by letter
- Discuss your findings with the patient and agree common ground. Where appropriate, discuss also with relatives

SECONDARY NON-ORGANIC DISORDERS

DEFINITION

Adjustment disorders, anxiety disorders and depressive disorders are the commonest psychological reaction to physical illnesses, both acute and chronic.

CLINICAL FEATURES

See pages 160 and 161 for a discussion of anxiety and depressive disorders. Adjustment disorders (ICD-10 F43.2) are periods of subjective distress and emotional disturbance usually interfering with social functioning and performance, arising in a period of adaptation to a significant life change or stressful event. They can take the form of a brief or prolonged depressive reaction, or a mixed anxiety and depressive reaction, or occur with predominant disturbance of conduct and emotions or of conduct alone. Onset is within 1 month of the stressor.

EPIDEMIOLOGY

Adjustment disorders are the commonest psychological reaction to physical illnesses, both acute and chronic.

Anxiety disorders have a prevalence of 5–20% among general hospital patients.

Affective disorders can be diagnosed in 20–30% of new medical outpatients.

The relationship of psychiatric comorbidity to the outcome of a physical disorder is unclear, some workers suggesting that psychiatric disorder slows recovery from physical illness and some suggesting that those patients with more serious physical illnesses are more likely to be depressed than those with milder conditions. A proportion of affective disorders persist after discharge, especially in patients with a past psychiatric history.

BASIC SCIENCES

A period of psychological readjustment following a physical illness or surgery is a normal and early response but it has been suggested that prolonged and maladaptive adjustment reactions are associated with poorer long-term outcome of the physical condition. Most studies show that the associations of psychological disorders in the physically ill are similar to those in the non-physically ill. Such variables as life events, poor social support, lack of 'mastery' and previous psychiatric history have all been implicated. Although the type and severity of the physical illness is indeed relevant, it is not as important a variable as one might expect.

DIFFERENTIAL DIAGNOSIS

- Appropriate response to illness or mental illness?
- Pre-existing or new mental illness?

Some common medical causes of secondary anxiety and depressive disorders:

CARDIOVASCULAR

- Myocardial infarction
- Heart failure
- Dysrhythmias

- **RESPIRATORY**
  - Asthma
  - Chronic obstructive airways disease
  - Respiratory failure
- **GASTROINTESTINAL**
  - Inflammatory bowel disease
  - Peptic ulceration
- **NEUROLOGICAL**
  - Cerebrovascular disorders
  - Multiple sclerosis
  - Head injury
  - Epilepsy
- **ENDOCRINE/METABOLIC**
  - Electrolyte imbalance
  - Hypoglycaemia
  - Thyroid disease
  - Cushing's disease
  - Addison's disease
  - Parathyroid disease
  - Pituitary disorders
- **INFECTIVE**
  - HIV with and without AIDS
  - Epstein–Barr virus
  - Hepatitis
  - Syphilis
- **DRUGS**
  - Sympathomimetics and their withdrawal
  - Sedatives and their withdrawal
  - Steroids
  - Antihypertensives
  - Beta-blockers
  - Analgesics
  - L-dopa

MANAGEMENT

Physical

Benzodiazepines may be indicated for the short-term management of anxiety. If they are initiated, it should be ensured that they are not continued indefinitely. If the patient meets criteria for a major depressive disorder, an antidepressant should be considered. Appropriate doses should be used bearing in mind the patient's physical condition and the actions and side-effect profile of the drug to be used. See the section on mood disorders on page 154. Look for prescribed medications that may produce psychological symptoms.

Psychological

Simple explanation can go a long way. The indications for specific psychological therapies are discussed on page 235. Consideration should be given to the need for referral to specific counselling agencies either within the hospital or in the community.

Social

What is the most appropriate environment in which to manage the patient? Should other agencies be involved to address concerns about accommodation, family, pets, finances?

PROGNOSIS

The majority of adjustment reactions are self-limiting. The naturalistic outcome of mood and anxiety disorders is not as favourable as once thought: up to one-third remain cases at 1 year without effective treatment, emphasizing the need for intervention.

DELIRIUM

DEFINITION

This organic syndrome is the final common pathway for a wide range of pathologies. It is characterized by waxing and waning global disturbances of consciousness and attention, cognition, psychomotor activity, the sleep–wake cycle, and affect.

CLINICAL FEATURES

The rapidly fluctuating course of delirium is often characteristic. There may be lucid intervals. Core symptoms are:

- **IMPAIRMENT OF CONSCIOUSNESS AND ATTENTION**, characteristically in a waxing and waning fashion and with easy distractibility
- **GLOBAL DISTURBANCE OF COGNITION**
  This may involve disorientation in time and place (rarely person), memory, registration of new material, delusions, illusions, hallucinations and misperceptions and perceptual disturbances in any sensory modality. Visual disturbances, illusions and hallucinations are relatively common
- **PSYCHOMOTOR DISTURBANCES**
  The patient may be overactive (as in delirium tremens) or underactive (as an elderly person with organ failure may sometimes be)
- **EMOTIONAL DISTURBANCES**
  At times the person may be elated, anxious, depressed, hostile, perplexed or any other emotion

NEUROLOGICAL FEATURES

For example, dysphasia, dysgraphia, constructional apraxia, abnormalities of gait, tremor, myoclonus, changes in reflexes and muscle tone

EPIDEMIOLOGY

Delirium is associated with many physical illnesses, especially infective and metabolic conditions, any disorders of the central nervous system, substance abuse, prescribed drug taking and end-organ failure. Such illnesses are also common in certain environments associated with under- or overstimulation, such as intensive care (30% of patients versus 10% on medical wards). Overall prevalence estimates among general hospital populations suggest that between one-quarter and one-third of patients have intellectual impairment. By and large, studies do not differentiate between acute, chronic and acute-on-chronic organic conditions, even although the early identification of acute organic states is crucial because of the need to treat the underlying condition and the high associated mortality rate. There is a high risk of delirium in association with increasing age, pre-existing brain disease, substance abuse, burns and HIV-related disorders.

BASIC SCIENCES

Diverse aetiologies result in a similar clinical picture. Classically, the causes are infective, metabolic, anoxic and endocrine conditions, prescribed drugs, substance abuse, diseases of the central nervous system and end-organ failure. Among the hospitalized elderly the cause may not be established in up to 20%. Male attenders at A & E departments and inpatients on orthopaedic, surgical and medical wards show a high prevalence of alcohol problems. Many such patients have alcohol-related conditions but the prevalence of alcohol problems is also high among patients whose current illness is not directly alcohol-related, most studies finding that approximately 20–25% of acute hospital admissions are related to alcohol. Thus acute intoxication and withdrawal are common.

DIFFERENTIAL DIAGNOSIS

The differential diagnoses to be considered are extensive. It is important to focus on easily reversible causes or conditions that will rapidly progress without intervention, such as Wernicke's encephalopathy.

CARDIOVASCULAR

Cardiac failure, hypovolaemia or hypoperfusion, myocardial infarction, dysrhythmias, hypertensive encephalopathy

RESPIRATORY

Respiratory failure, anoxia from any cause (remember carbon monoxide poisoning), pulmonary embolus

- **NEUROLOGICAL**
  Cerebrovascular accident, space-occupying lesion from any cause, especially an intracranial bleed. Multiple sclerosis, Parkinson's disease. Epileptic: postictal
- **METABOLIC/ENDOCRINE**
  Hypoglycaemia
- **INFECTIONS**
  Urinary tract infection, pneumonia, meningitis, encephalitis, atypical infections in the immunocompromised patient, abscess
- **SUBSTANCE ABUSE**
  Alcohol: either intoxication or withdrawal. Poisons
- **PRESCRIBED DRUGS**
  Either at normal or excess dose. Anticholinergic drugs, antibiotics, analgesics, antiparkinsonian drugs, anticonvulsants, cardiovascular drugs, psychotropic drugs, sympathomimetics, CNS depressants, cimetidine. Any drug in the elderly should come under suspicion
- **NUTRITIONAL**
  Thiamine, B_{12}, folate and niacin deficiencies. Look particularly for Wernicke's encephalopathy: delirium, ophthalmoplegia (lateral gaze palsy), nystagmus, ataxia and peripheral neuropathy
- **MALIGNANCY**
  Metastatic or non-metastatic complications
- **TRAUMA**
  Head injury, postoperative, burns, major trauma
- **DEMENTIA**
  Usually preserved consciousness and insidious onset
- **OTHER PSYCHIATRIC**
  Schizophrenia, schizotypal and delusional disorders, mood disorders particularly mania, dissociative disorders, Ganser's syndrome, malingering, sensory deprivation

MANAGEMENT

Physical

Pay particular attention to history and examination. A more thorough cognitive state examination may be necessary. Consider using the Mini Mental State Examination (MMSE). Also look at current management and investigations: full blood count, urea and electrolytes, liver function tests, calcium, alkaline phosphatase, thyroid function tests, blood gases, blood cultures, lumbar puncture, B_{12}, folate, imaging, psychometric testing. The management then becomes the treatment of the underlying cause.

In the case of agitation, opinions differ as to the drug of choice. Many use haloperidol for its relative lack of anticholinergic and hypotensive effects. However, it has extrapyramidal side-effects. The lowest effective dose should be used, much lower than for acute psychosis, probably titrating the patient in 500 μg doses by an appropriate route. Some also use benzodiazepines for agitation.

Psychological

Generally speaking, staff in intensive-care settings are highly skilled at communicating with delirious patients and know what to do. The aim is to avoid over- or understimulation through the use of acceptable lighting levels with clear day/night distinctions and television or other stimuli if appropriate. Clear simple explanations and reassurance for the patient are important.

PROGNOSIS

Often dependent upon prognosis of the underlying physical condition.

SOMATIZATION

DEFINITION

Somatization is best understood as a process rather than a disease and is the most common way for psychiatric disorders to present in non-psychiatric settings as medically unexplained physical symptoms. Somatic symptoms as part of an affective disorder are much more common than somatoform disorder or conversion disorder.

CLINICAL FEATURES

MEDICALLY UNEXPLAINED SOMATIC SYMPTOMS

These are common. Recurrent presentation of medically unexplained physical symptoms with persistent requests for further investigation despite reassurance and negative findings. Comorbid physical disorders might account for the symptoms. The liaison psychiatrist may often be asked to see such patients. There will often be a mood disorder present.

SOMATIZATION DISORDER

Also known in the USA as Briquet's syndrome or Briquet's hysteria, this disorder is much less common. It has been criticized as a pejorative diagnosis made by physicians about predominantly female patients they dislike. The sufferer should be less than 30 years old at onset, have a 'dramatic, complex' medical history and have 25 symptoms in nine groups from a list of 65 in 10 groups covering all systems.

PAIN DISORDER

Formerly called somatoform pain disorder in the *Diagnostic and Statistical*

Manual of Mental Disorders, 3rd edn (revised) (DSM-III-R), the diagnosis was rarely used. However, pain is a frequent complaint. It is unhelpful to distinguish between functional and organic pain. In patients with chronic pain it is more helpful to look for evidence of depression, anxiety, somatization, conversion, malingering and factitious disorder.

DISSOCIATIVE (CONVERSION) DISORDER

Practically this involves a loss or alteration of function suggestive of a physical, usually neurological, condition. Typical examples are paralysis, changes in consciousness, fits, abnormal gait, tremor or aphonia. It may also involve sensory changes such as blindness or anaesthesia.

EPIDEMIOLOGY

Somatic symptoms are very common: 64% of a consecutive series of 94 referrals to a cardiology clinic with chest pain had no underlying physical illness. Certain groups are known to be at particular high risk – those with unexplained somatic symptoms such as irritable bowel, chronic fatigue, facial pain and so on. The range of symptoms is large and somatization occurs in all medical settings. The primary psychiatric diagnosis in most cases is primary affective disorder although a significant majority are suffering from somatoform, dissociative or factitious disorders.

Somatization disorder is reported to have a community prevalence of between 0.03% and 0.4% in the USA. In health-care settings it is reported much more frequently in women (20:1). There are strong associations with other psychiatric disorders, mainly mood, substance abuse and personality disorders. Some research has suggested that first-degree male relatives have increased rates of personality disorder and substance abuse and female relatives have high rates of somatization.

The epidemiology of pain disorder is not clear.

Dissociative (conversion) disorders have been around for a long time as hysteria, yet surprisingly little is known about their epidemiology. They are commoner in women than men. Between 15 and 33% go on to have a physical disorder diagnosed and 33% have a mood disorder at follow-up.

BASIC SCIENCES

Dissociative (conversion) disorder in the guise of hysteria was originally assumed to be the manifestation of repressed emotions and feelings. The conversion of anxiety/conflicts to physical symptoms was thought to reduce anxiety about the conflict producing primary gain. The attention of others gives secondary gain. There is no evidence of twin-pair concordance but a slightly higher incidence in first-degree relatives is observed. Abnormal illness behaviour is a useful framework within which to consider the nature of somatization. There is some evidence that life events can precipitate somatization.

DIFFERENTIAL DIAGNOSIS

- **PHYSICAL DISORDER**
  Either alone or with comorbid psychiatric disorder
- **PSYCHIATRIC DISORDER**
  Mood disorder, anxiety disorder, adjustment disorder, hypochondriasis, personality disorder, delirium, psychosis
- **MALINGERING, FACTITIOUS DISORDER (MUNCHAUSEN SYNDROME)**

MANAGEMENT[1]

Physical

Whether in clinic or inpatient settings, the first step is to review the history, examinations and investigations for evidence of a physical disorder. Otherwise the physical management is of the underlying psychiatric disorder. However, this is unlikely to be achieved before establishing a rapport with the patient.

Psychological

It is vitally important to take the patient's complaints seriously. Establish a rapport with the patient and explain why they are being seen by a psychiatrist. Once a relationship is established it may be helpful to note that the person may be distressed by their symptoms and then ask screening questions about mood and the patient's views on aetiology. The idea is to perform the least number of investigations possible and to then begin to re-attribute the symptoms to allow consideration of psychological factors. Specific psychological therapies have been demonstrated to be effective for some somatic conditions, e.g. irritable bowel syndrome.

Social

Attention should be paid to the rewards the patient gains from their illness behaviour and the response of the person's network, both professional and family. What the person stands to lose by changing should also be considered.

PROGNOSIS

Untreated somatization disorder involves the patient in unnecessary treatments and investigations. Dissociative disorders have a good prognosis if they have an acute onset and the nature of the conflict/life event is clear and resolvable. Poor prognosis is associated with underlying personality disorder and lack of motivation to change.

ONCOLOGY

PSYCHIATRIC PRESENTATIONS

- Adjustment disorders
- Bereavement reactions
- Anxiety disorders
- Mood disorders: manic and depressive states
- Suicidality
- Paranoid states
- Delirium
- Substance abuse

Much of the psychiatric morbidity associated with cancer, as with other illnesses, goes unrecognized and untreated. Although exact prevalence data are unavailable it is known that mastectomy, chemotherapy and colostomy are associated with substantial psychiatric morbidity. As in other physical illnesses, non-psychotic syndromes such as anxiety and depression predominate. Rates for psychiatric referral and treatment are higher than is usually found in medical and surgical wards, oncology being an area where physicians increasingly recognize the importance of attending to the patient's psychosocial wellbeing. One area of specific interest is the increasing body of evidence showing that in breast cancer a patient's coping style may influence the outcome of the malignancy. Cognitive behavioural treatments have been designed to optimize patients' coping styles. There are often specialist staff attached to oncology services who can offer excellent support. There is a growing body of evidence that treatment of mood disorders, even in terminal care settings, can improve quality of life.

THE DYING PATIENT

A further liaison function for the psychiatrist is to work with the terminally ill and the medical and surgical teams who care for them. The diagnosis of terminal illness or malignancy initiates the stages of grieving and coming to terms with the loss of aspirations, health and interpersonal relationships with family and friends. The reactions of patients vary from denial (normal, as in the early stages of grief) to anxiety states, minor depression and severe depressive states. Those with peripheral cerebral/lung metastases may also suffer organic confusional states. Delirium in the absence of cerebral metastases is a well-known paraneoplastic phenomenon.

The role of the psychiatrist is to facilitate abnormal grief from self-limiting anxiety states (adjustment reactions), facilitate communication between the patient and relatives or friends, assess mood states and consider interventions such as antidepressant medication or cognitive therapy. Problem-solving and anxiety management techniques are of value and enable the patient to plan the remaining days as well as take care of 'unfinished business' in terms of relationships and financial provision for survivors.

REACTIONS OF THE DYING PATIENT

- Denial
- Anger
- Bargaining
- Anxiety and depression
- More realistic acceptance

Certain criteria used in the diagnosis of depression need careful evaluation in the terminally ill patient in view of their occurrence in malignancy. Thus fatigue, lack of energy, poor concentration, preoccupation with death and sleep disturbance, non-recognition and poor treatment of depression in the terminally ill may compromise their ability to arrange final plans for themselves and their families. Rating scales are of value but cut-off score should invariably be higher for population-based instruments. The Hospital Anxiety and Depression Scale (HADS) has been successfully used.

The active management should be reviewed frequently and altered if unsuccessful. Interpersonal difficulties, social isolation, poverty, rapidly declining ability to care for self and physical disability all contribute. The treatments (cytotoxics, radiotherapy) themselves are difficult and uncomfortable and uncertainty about the prognosis around treatment cycles will compound the 'understandable' reactions. Explain carefully the purpose of medication, the adverse-effect profile and the need to review treatment, and do deliver supportive psychotherapy or specifically target depressive symptoms with cognitive therapy. Be aware of potential interactions of prescribed psychotropic drugs, physical illness in malignancy and cytotoxic drugs. Doses may need to be reduced. Assess suicide risk thoroughly. Much of the work involves supportive psychotherapy.

OBSTETRICS AND GYNAECOLOGY

PSYCHIATRIC PRESENTATIONS IN OBSTETRICS

ANTENATAL

- Depression or deliberate self harm
- Acute stress reactions or adjustment disorders relating to fetal abnormality, still birth, perinatal death
- Post-traumatic stress disorder from difficult labour
- Phobia of needles or labour (tocophobia)
- Substance misuse in pregnancy

POSTNATAL

- Postpartum blues
- Puerperal psychosis
- Postnatal depression
- Recurrence/exacerbation of pre-existing mental illness

PSYCHIATRIC PRESENTATIONS IN GYNAECOLOGY

- Premenstrual syndrome (premenstrual dysphoric disorder – DSM-IV)
- Acute stress reactions or adjustment disorder related to miscarriage, termination of pregnancy, infertility and cancer
- Psychosexual problems, e.g. vaginismus
- Psychological sequelae of gynaecological disease, e.g. endometriosis, polycystic ovarian disease
- Mood changes related to the menopause
- Chronic pelvic pain

MANAGEMENT OF OBSTETRIC AND GYNAECOLOGY REFERRALS

Emotional distress and anxiety are common and often normal responses to pregnancy loss or gynaecological symptoms. Patients require sensitive explanations, empathy, information and support. Occasionally, the intensity of a woman's reaction or frequency of help-seeking behaviour becomes extreme and on such occasions a psychiatrist may be asked to provide an opinion. It is important in assessing such patients to consider significant issues in the personal history (e.g. past losses, guilt over past abortions, childhood sexual abuse) and relevant personality issues.

Adjustment disorders often respond to brief psychosocial support and counselling but, if symptoms are protracted or severe, antidepressant medication or a structured cognitive behavioural therapy approach may be required.

Premenstrual syndrome, also known as premenstrual dysphoric disorder (DSM-IV), is diagnosed when mood changes (lability, irritability), behavioural changes (hypersomnia, food cravings) and physical symptoms (breast tenderness, swelling) occurring in the last week of the menstrual cycle impact on social functioning. Differential diagnosis is of a chronic or recurrent depressive disorder – in these cases the symptoms persist after the menses. Fluoxetine is currently the only antidepressant to have a licence to treat this condition. Other treatments include evening primrose oil and vitamin B_6.

MENTAL ILLNESS IN PREGNANCY

Depression in pregnancy is more commonly seen in younger women with more children, whereas postpartum depression shows no association with age, number of children or educational status. Depression arising in later pregnancy has a worse prognosis than first-trimester depression and is a risk factor for subsequent postnatal mental illness.

Drug treatment should be avoided in pregnancy unless the likely benefits to the mother outweigh the risks to the fetus. The tricyclics (amitriptyline, imipramine) are the drugs of choice for the treatment of depression in pregnancy, because of their safety record. Cumulative data on fluoxetine have shown no increased incidence of fetal abnormalities or long-term neurodevelopmental problems and it can be used if the patient can not tolerate tricyclic antidepressants. Newer antidepressants such as venlafaxine should be avoided unless there are extreme clinical benefits, e.g. treatment resistance with other antidepressants. ECT is relatively safe for severe depression and mania occurring in pregnancy.

POSTNATAL MENTAL ILLNESS

Postnatal mental illness, particularly depression, is common but generally presents in the community after discharge from the maternity unit.

Postpartum blues is characterized by emotional lability and anxiety occurring on the third to fifth postpartum day. It should be considered a normal phenomenon occurring in 50% of women. It is important to differentiate this from early-onset severe depression or puerperal psychosis.

Puerperal psychosis is a rare (1 per 1000) disorder occurring acutely within the first few weeks after birth (in most cases the onset will occur between the third and the 14th days). The aetiology is unknown but opinion generally favours a biological rather than a psychosocial cause. Some authors have postulated a hypersensitivity to oestrogen withdrawal affecting dopamine receptors in genetically determined women. The clinical picture is suggestive of an affective disorder. Women with a history of bipolar affective disorder or a family history of affective disorder are most at risk and have a 30–50% chance of recurrence in subsequent pregnancies. Other risk factors include a first birth (relative risk 2), and some studies report higher incidences following caesarean section.

Special features in the psychopathology include:

- Prodromal symptoms of irritability, restlessness, sleeplessness and incongruent mood
- A similar presentation to an acute organic confusional state, e.g. a fluctuating clouding of consciousness with misinterpretation of visual stimuli
- Delusions of grandeur or persecution with associated auditory and visual hallucination
- Abnormal beliefs regarding the baby, e.g. evil in baby, death of baby and substitution of impostor.

Puerperal psychosis should be treated as an acute psychiatric emergency. The presentation in the acute stage can fluctuate and the condition of the woman may rapidly deteriorate. In most cases the mother will require admission. A risk assessment should include the risk of harm to the baby by the mother (neglect and physical abuse) and to the mother by suicide or recklessness.

The differential diagnosis includes acute delirium secondary to septicaemia or breast abscess, and posteclamptic psychosis.

Ideally, the mother should be admitted with her baby to a specialist mother and baby unit. Separation can prolong the episode and cause interruption to the bonding process. Treatment may include antipsychotic medication, mood stabilizers and antidepressants. Nursing care will focus on assessing and strengthening the mother–infant bond. Research on secondary prevention with oestrogen patches indicates some effectiveness, although the total evidence is limited.

POSTNATAL DEPRESSION

In contrast to puerperal psychosis the aetiology of postnatal depression is thought to be psychosocial rather than biological. Vulnerability factors include a poor marital relationship, a history of psychiatric illness, lack of a confidante and high levels of anxiety in pregnancy. Adverse life events, poor social circumstances and a history of severe 'baby blues' and depression in pregnancy increases the risk. No abnormality in the hormone profile has been found, although thyroid antibodies and thyroid function should be tested.

The peak onset is between 4 and 6 weeks after delivery, with more severe episodes occurring early. The illness may run an insidious course and may go undetected, with devastating consequences for the mother's wellbeing and her relationships, including bonding and attachment difficulties with her infant. The adverse effects of a depressed mother on the child are seen particularly in boys, who may show behavioural problems and emotional difficulties into late childhood. Routine screening using the Edinburgh Postnatal Self-report Questionnaire at the 6-week check is now recommended.

Randomized control studies have demonstrated the effectiveness of brief directive counselling. Some health visitors are trained to administer 'listening visits' using brief problem-solving approaches. Postnatal support groups and voluntary agencies also have an important part to play in the management of these women. Other treatments include antidepressant drugs. Tricyclics can be prescribed to mothers who are breast-feeding provided the baby is full-term and healthy. There is a lack of evidence to support the use of progesterone or oestrogen, although these are commonly prescribed by obstetricians and general practitioners.

TERMINATION AND MISCARRIAGE

Of women in the post-termination period, 10% develop depression or anxiety; psychosis is rare.[3]

It is now commonplace to offer brief counselling before termination of pregnancy. This primary preventive strategy has been shown to reduce the likelihood of subsequent psychiatric complications. Psychiatric problems are more common following miscarriage and stillbirth and a well-designed randomized controlled study of prompt bereavement counselling following perinatal deaths backed up by appropriate obstetric support and advice demonstrated that intervention was effective in reducing psychiatric complications at 6 months.

Risk factors: past psychiatric history, poor social support, multiparity, fetal abnormality, belonging to groups that are opposed to termination, younger age group. Most reactions last less than 3 months. Two-thirds of women have had previous psychiatric care. Guilt is present in one-third of women before termination and in less than 10% of them at 2 years. There are conflicting estimates of prevalence of chronic cases, ranging from one-third at 6 months to 20% at 1–2 years.

HIV INFECTION AND AIDS

PSYCHIATRIC PRESENTATIONS

- **Adjustment disorders**
- **Bereavement reactions**
- **Anxiety disorders (including the worried well)**
- **Mood disorders**
- **Organic disorders including:**
  - Delirium
  - Secondary brain infection
  - HIV dementia

EPIDEMIOLOGY

Highest rates of HIV infection are seen in the developing world, where the prevalence in some areas is as high as 50% of the adult population. Most infections in the UK are acquired through unprotected sexual intercourse (many through contact abroad). Needle-sharing has become less common among drug users, although there is still an increased prevalence of HIV and hepatitis B among intravenous drug users.

Blood for HIV testing should never be taken without full consent and pre- and post-test counselling should be given.

The psychiatric consequences of a diagnosis include psychological reactions and neuropsychiatric complications. HIV-positive people have a high risk of suicide and deliberate self harm. This is highest in patients with previous depression, personality disorder and substance misuse.

Significant HIV-related cognitive impairment usually occurs where significant immunosuppression is present. Early organic brain impairment can present as a functional psychosis, commonly hypomania or a paranoid psychosis. Cognitive testing reveals impaired short-term memory, concentration and psychomotor retardation. Up to 65% of hospitalized AIDS patients have some degree of cognitive impairment but only 10–15% will develop full dementia. HIV dementia (HIV encephalopathy) causes frontal lobe dysfunction with associated personality changes, apathy and social withdrawal. Ataxia, hypertonia and hyper-reflexia may be present on physical examination. Severe dementia occurs as a late complication of the disease and is an AIDS-defining disorder. Opportunistic infections such as toxoplasmosis and lymphoma can present with acute organic brain syndromes with focal neurological signs caused by space-occupying lesions.

MANAGEMENT

Immediate management usually focuses on the assessment and management of behavioural problems and neuropsychiatric states (delirium, dementia). HIV services are being established to meet the special needs of HIV-positive patients who have minor anxiety and depressive reactions as well as those developing severe mental illness. Recent evidence indicates that the severely mentally ill (schizophrenia and bipolar disorder) are at high risk of developing HIV because of high-risk sexual behaviour, usually unprotected sex. Well-integrated services include genitourinary assessments, medical liaison, counselling services and psychology and psychiatric input aimed at primary, secondary and tertiary prevention. Hospice care for the terminally ill and family support are also necessary components. Some groups (African women, children) need further specialist services that can engage them and provide a service suited to their unique profile of needs.

PSYCHOLOGICAL AND EMOTIONAL PROBLEMS AMONG RELATIVES

- **Bereavement reactions**
- **Adjustment disorders**
- **Mood disorders**

The physical illness of a family member can have serious repercussions for other family members that go beyond practical considerations of financial hardship, the burden of caring for a sick relative and uncertainty about prognosis. Following the death of the patient, relatives have to cope with bereavement and readjustment. Following myocardial infarction, spouses experience similar levels of psychological distress to the patient. During rehabilitation and when looking after a chronically ill, disabled or dying patient, the carer often experiences considerable psychological distress. Among the elderly, when one partner is admitted to hospital, the other may not be able to function alone if the sick person was the primary carer for the couple. The liaison psychiatrist is well placed to suggest that staff attend to this area.

The most important strategy involves the provision of adequate and comprehensible information, support and attention given at the appropriate time. Generally, a psychiatrist is only involved in this process when a relative becomes acutely disturbed. However, psychiatrists have an important role to play in educating students and staff in this process, a strategy that could also have useful public relations benefits for the liaison psychiatric team.

PSYCHOLOGICAL AND EMOTIONAL PROBLEMS AMONG STAFF

Recent studies among junior hospital doctors have highlighted something that has been known for a long time – working in hospitals is a stressful experience. Levels of anxiety and depression among doctors are high and rates of alcohol and drug abuse and self-harm are increased in the medical profession. Over 30% of junior doctors experience significant psychological distress. Rates are even higher among female house officers, 46% of whom were significantly depressed in one study. Within hospitals, certain areas, such as intensive care units, oncology, paediatric departments and renal dialysis units, are recognized as being particularly stressful. Health professionals are generally poor at seeking help for their own mental health problems. Most hospitals have occupational health departments and in some larger hospitals members of the liaison team are involved in the service provided. Opportunities for primary prevention exist in the provision of support and guidance for staff, either formally in groups or by easy access to services. At present, little training or teaching is provided for medical students on how to recognize symptoms in themselves and the climate does not exist in which sufferers feel comfortable admitting their symptoms and seeking help. There is a national counselling service for sick doctors. Local initiatives depend on the occupational health service and acceptance of the psychiatrist and role of the liaison team.

REFERENCES

1. Creed F, Mayou R, Hopkins A, ed. Medical symptoms not explained by organic disease. London: Gaskell, 1992.
2. Cox JL, Holden JM, Sagovsky R et al. Detection of postnatal depression: development of a 10 item Edinburgh Postnatal Depression Scale. Br J Psychiatry 1987: 160: 742–749.
3. Zolese G, Blacker CV. The psychological consequences of therapeutic abortion. Br J Psychiatry 1992; 160: 742–749.
4. Everall IP. Neuropsychiatric aspects of HIV infection. J Neurol Neurosurg Psychiatry 1995: 58: 399–402.

SECTION VI

Comprehensive Local Services

COMMUNITY CARE LEGISLATION

The White Paper *Caring for People* (1989) set out the policy, while the NHS and Community Care Act 1990 set out the legal framework. Acts of Parliament under which community care services are defined for the purposes of the NHS and Community Care Act are listed below.

- **NATIONAL ASSISTANCE ACT 1948**
  Part III section 21(1) as amended by the NHS and Community Care Act states that: 'It shall be the duty of every local authority to provide for persons who, by reason of age, illness, disability or any other circumstances are in need of care and attention which is not otherwise available to them'
- **HEALTH SERVICES AND PUBLIC HEALTH ACT 1968**
  Section 45(1) of this Act gives local authorities powers to make arrangements to promote the welfare of old people
- **NATIONAL HEALTH SERVICE ACT 1977**
  Schedule 8, paragraph 3(1) states that every local authority should provide adequate help for households where a person is 'suffering from illness, lying in, an expectant mother, aged, handicapped...'. It also gives powers to local authorities to provide services for people who are physically or mentally ill, such as day services
- **MENTAL HEALTH ACT 1983**
  Section 117 imposes a duty of aftercare for certain patients by health authorities and social services. The Care Programme Approach (1991) extends that to all persons in contact with secondary-care services. Supervised discharges apply to some persons who have been detained in hospital under the Mental Health Act

MODERNISING MENTAL HEALTH SERVICES

The White Paper *Modernising Mental Health Services* (1999) began from the position that community care had failed. It then set out a vision for 'safe, sound and supportive' mental health services and identified seven priority areas for development:

- Strengthening comprehensive care
- Providing 24 hour access to services
- Developing, training and recruiting staff with the skills and motivation to deliver modern services
- Improving the planning and commissioning of services
- Developing partnership working
- Improving the use of information technology
- Developing mental health promotion.

THE NATIONAL SERVICE FRAMEWORK

The national service framework for mental health services (1999) was one of the first three service frameworks to be published, along with cardiovascular disease and cancer. It set out seven standards against which all mental health services should be measured. The implementation of the standards is tightly performance-managed. These seven standards are intended to provide a framework for delivering a high-quality, comprehensive mental health service that is equitable and locally accountable.

THE SEVEN STANDARDS

- **MENTAL HEALTH PROMOTION: health and social services should promote mental health for all, working with individuals and communities to combat discrimination against individuals and groups with mental health problems and promote their social inclusion**
- **Any service user who contacts their primary health-care team with a common mental health problem should have their mental health needs identified and assessed and be offered effective treatments, including referral to specialist services for further assessment, treatment and care if they require it**
- **Any individual with a common mental health problem should be able to make contact round the clock with the local services necessary to meet their needs and receive adequate care, and be able to use NHS Direct, as it develops, for first-level advice and referral on to specialist helplines or to local services**
- **All mental health service users on the care programme approach (CPA) should:**
  - Receive care that optimizes engagement, prevents or anticipates crisis, and reduces risk
  - Have a copy of a written care plan that: includes the action to be taken in a crisis by the service user, their carer and their care coordinator; specifically advises their GP how they should respond if the service user needs additional help; and is regularly reviewed by their care coordinator
  - Be able to access services 24 hours a day, 365 days a year
- **Each service user who is assessed as requiring a period of care away from their home should have timely access to an appropriate hospital bed or alternative bed or place, which is in the least restrictive environment consistent with the need to protect them and the public, and as close to home as possible. They should also have a copy of a written aftercare plan, agreed on discharge, which sets out the care and rehabilitation to be provided, identifies the care coordinator and specifies the action to be taken in a crisis**

- **All individuals who provide regular and substantial care for a person on the CPA should have an assessment of their caring, physical and mental health needs, repeated on at least an annual basis, and have their own written care plan, which is given to them and implemented in discussion with them**
- **Preventing suicide: local health and social care agencies should prevent suicide by implementing standards 1–6 above and, in addition: support local prison staff in preventing suicide among prisoners; ensure that staff are competent to assess the risk of suicide among individuals at greatest risk; and develop local systems for suicide audit to learn lessons and take any necessary action**

COMPONENTS OF A COMPREHENSIVE LOCAL SERVICE

A typical range of service settings for adults is described below. 24-hour access to a range of services is a core concept of the national service framework.

Table 4 Components of a local framework

	Acute/emergency care	Rehabilitation/ continuing care
Home-based	Early intervention Intensive home support Emergency duty teams Sector teams	Assertive outreach teams Domiciliary services Keyworkers Care management
Day care	Day hospitals	Drop-in centres Support groups Employment schemes Day care
Residential	Crisis accommodation Acute units Local secure units	Ordinary housing support Unstaffed group homes Adult placement schemes Residential care homes Mental nursing homes 24-hour NHS accommodation Medium-security units High-security units

THE REVISED CARE PROGRAMME APPROACH

The revised CPA involves a number of elements:

Table 5 Relationships between CPA and other legislation and guidance[7,8]

Legislation/guidance	Target group
Care programme approach (CPA)	All people accepted by specialist psychiatric services
Care management	People on CPA with related social-care needs
Supervision register	People on CPA with severe mental illness who may be a serious risk to self or others
Section 117 aftercare	People discharged after admission under sections 3, 37, 47, 48 of the Mental Health Act 1983 (MHA). CPA also applies. Supervision register may apply
Guardianship	People placed on guardianship order under MHA. CPA applies. Section 117 and supervision register may apply
Supervised discharge	Some people who have been detained under MHA while in hospital. All subject to section 117 and CPA. Many will be on supervision register

- **All persons referred to secondary services should have:**
  - A systematic *assessment* of health and social care needs
  - An agreed *care plan*
  - Allocation of a *keyworker*
  - Regular *review* of progress
  - A *tiered* approach reflecting level of need and service involvement
  - A CPA *register*

SECTORIZATION

More than 80% of psychiatric services in the UK are sectorized. The ideal population size is less than 50 000, depending on needs, demographics and services. Boundaries may be determined by GP practice, electoral ward, or health or local authority borders. Attempts are now being made to ensure that all agencies have coterminous boundaries. Mental health services must integrate with other local services and agencies.

NEEDS ASSESSMENT

Need is the concept that provides a link between a problem and an intervention for that problem. It is a measure of the problem and can be individual- or population-based. For an individual it can be rated by the patient, the carer or the health professional and involves a direct assessment of an individual's health. In the individual setting a need is only said to exist if there is a problem for which there is an available and accepted intervention. However, where disability exists there may be problem areas for which there are no known or readily available interventions; heated debate often serves to highlight the fact that a patient's perception of need may not be that of the professionals. For professionals, needs assessment attempts to individualize care in a systematic way and also enables the amount of health or illness to be measured in intervention terms. Needs assessment schedules[3,4] attempt to include questions about areas of need in the population for which the questionnaire was designed. It is unlikely that all populations will have the same profile of needs, although a core of needs (housing, benefits, physical health, etc.) is likely to be common to all populations. An aggregate of these individual assessments can give a broader picture of population needs but this process is costly in terms of time and manpower. Other ways to define need have included population-based studies using proxy measures of need as indicators of health or illness at a population level. These include medical information systems, social deprivation indices, service utilization and consumer/public opinion. Clinical care delivery is invariably limited by resources, and needs assessments serve as one way of monitoring resource use.

DOMICILIARY VISITS

- **Do** be clear why you are being asked to see the patient at home: Mental Health Act assessment, diagnostic uncertainty
- **Do** get as much background information as possible about current presentation and past history
- **Do** find out who else will be going
- **Do** say where you are going and who you will notify on your return
- **Do** take a mobile phone
- **Do** provide the referrer with verbal feedback at the time
- **Do** observe usual rules about personal safety in the person's home
- **Don't** visit alone if at all concerned
- **Do** take appropriate backup
- **Don't** over-react

PRIMARY-CARE PSYCHIATRY

PATHWAYS TO CARE

Of mental health problems, 95% are managed exclusively in primary care. At any one time, the average GP with 2000 patients has 300 with a diagnosed common mental disorder such as depression and anxiety. S/he will, on average, have around 10–15 patients with long-term psychotic mental illness.

Goldberg and Huxley's five levels and four filters on the pathways to psychiatric care[5] are described in Table 6.

Table 6 Goldberg and Huxley's steps on the pathway to psychiatric care[5]

Setting	Period prevalence (*n*/1000 at risk per year)
LEVEL 1: The community 1st filter – the decision to consult	260–315
LEVEL 2: Total primary-care morbidity 2nd filter – GP recognition	230
LEVEL 3: Conspicuous morbidity 3rd filter – the decision to refer	101.5
LEVEL 4: Mental illness services 4th filter – admission to psychiatric bed	20.8
LEVEL 5: Psychiatric inpatients	3.8–6.7

MODELS OF PRIMARY-CARE LIAISON

- Conventional outpatient clinic
- Informal meetings
- Shifted outpatients
- Consultation model
- Consultation–liaison model
- Collaborative model

Outpatient referral is the traditional route for obtaining a psychiatric opinion. GPs are clear what they want from such a service.

GENERAL PRACTITIONER REQUIREMENTS FROM OUTPATIENT SERVICES[6]

- Rapid assessment
- Shorter referral–appointment interval
- Better communication
- Clear management guidelines
- Statement of objectives of treatment

- Predicted response, complications and side-effects
- 6-monthly review plans for chronic patients
- Clearly stated role of GP and specialist in treatment
- Clarification of prescribing responsibilities
- Information booklets of therapies available

Over the last 25 years, more and more psychiatrists have established attachments to primary-care settings and a variety of liaison models have emerged. The 'shifted outpatients' is the most simple and common arrangement. The psychiatrist conducts his/her usual outpatient clinic, except that it takes place in a surgery. S/he can offer assessment, crisis intervention and 'hands on' management in the surgery. Patients often prefer to be seen in a primary-care setting and supervision of trainees is relatively easy. However, no research has been conducted to see whether this method helps the primary heath-care team to improve their own management skills. A major problem is providing this kind of service to all the practices in a sector. According to the 'consultation model', the psychiatrist advises the GP about management at regular intervals and also sees patients in primary care if required. In the 'consultation–liaison' model the psychiatrist attends practice meetings to discuss management problems with the primary health-care team. S/he may then see the patient, accompanied by the GP or other member of the primary health-care team or practice-attached community psychiatric nurse. More patients can be discussed in this way and there is better GP/psychiatrist contact. The collaborative approach is an extension of this model of working reflecting the increasing power of the GP in a primary-care-led NHS.

MANAGEMENT: A FRAMEWORK FOR CONSULTATION–LIAISON

- The referral: consider 'What for, why now, why worry, why change?'
- Diagnoses and personality
- Physical factors
- Somatization
- Psychological factors
- Social factors
- Level of functioning
- Medication
- Organization of care and network involved

The primary concern of the secondary-care team is persons with severe mental illness. The majority of persons with depression and anxiety can be managed exclusively in primary care. The psychiatrist has a role to support the primary health-care team in looking after this large group.

In addition to the patient-specific help suggested above, it might also be helpful to think about the practice's strategy for identifying patients with chronic anxiety and depression. A number of simple screening instruments exist that can facilitate this process. Above all, the main aim is to support the primary health-care team in their management of difficult cases by reviewing what the issues are, what has been tried so far and what other possibilities there are. This approach can be supplemented with teaching and educational materials for the primary health-care team.

PRIMARY CARE OF PERSONS WITH PSYCHOTIC MENTAL ILLNESS

- Clear lines of communication
- Clarity about responsibility
- Named keyworker
- Regular review

GPs are responsible under their terms of service for patients registered with them. The mental health team has responsibilities for persons in contact with services under the CPA. Some favour shared care. Above all, clear lines of communication are necessary.

REFERENCES

1. Department of Health. The health of the nation, 2nd ed. London: HMSO, 1994.
2. Department of Health. Our healthier nation. London: Department of Health, 1998.
3. Thornicroft G, Brewin C, Wing J. Measuring mental health needs. London: Gaskell, 1992.
4. Wing J. Meeting the needs of people with psychiatric disorders. Soc Psychiatry Psychiatr Epidemiol 1990; 25: 2–8.
5. Goldberg D, Huxley P. Common mental disorders: a bio-social model. London: Routledge, 1992: 15–30.
6. Strathdee G. Psychiatry and general practice – a psychiatric perspective. In: Pullen I, Wilkinson G, Wright A, Pereira Gray D, eds. Psychiatry and general practice today. London: Royal College of Psychiatrists and Royal College of General Practitioners, 1994: 22–35.
7. Department of Health. Modernising mental health services. London, Department of Health, 1999.
8. Department of Health. National service framework for mental illness. London, Department of Health, 1999.

SECTION VII

Special Topics

FORENSIC PSYCHIATRY

Forensic psychiatry is the psychiatry of mentally abnormal offenders and the legal aspects of psychiatry. This is intended to be a brief introduction to the subject that will direct the reader to larger works where further information can be found.

STRUCTURE OF THE SERVICE

Forensic psychiatry services are usually based in secure hospitals. There are three maximum-security (special) hospitals in England – Rampton, Broadmoor and Ashworth – and a larger number of medium-security units, with at least one of these for each regional health authority in England and Wales. A growing number of forensic psychiatrists are based in low-security units and some may work exclusively with community-based patients. Typically, other components may include a court liaison service or special links with the local police service. In general terms, a patient should not be admitted to a hospital that has a greater level of security than is required to manage the risk, and the special hospitals require that patients should not be admitted unless they fulfil the relevant criteria for detention in hospital under the Mental Health Act 1983 and pose 'a grave and immediate danger to the public'

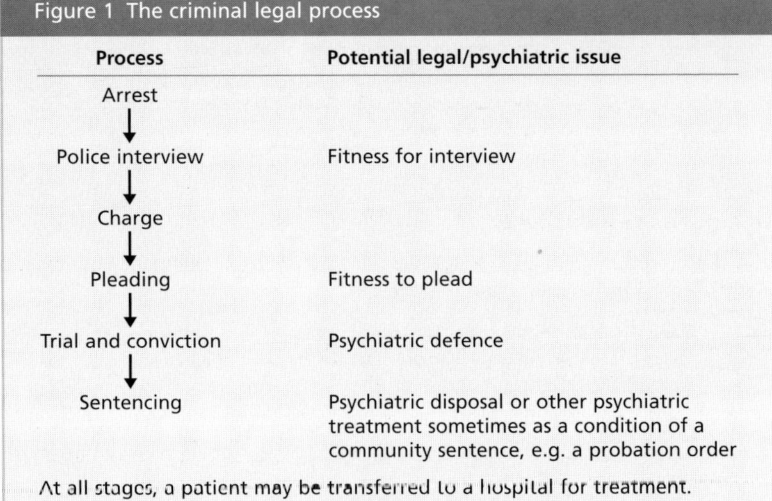

Figure 1 The criminal legal process

Process	Potential legal/psychiatric issue
Arrest ↓	
Police interview ↓	Fitness for interview
Charge ↓	
Pleading ↓	Fitness to plead
Trial and conviction ↓	Psychiatric defence
Sentencing	Psychiatric disposal or other psychiatric treatment sometimes as a condition of a community sentence, e.g. a probation order

At all stages, a patient may be transferred to a hospital for treatment. Prior to sentencing a person may be either remanded into custody (i.e. prison), remanded to hospital for a report, or bailed. A defendant may be bailed to an address in the community, a hostel or a hospital. Breaching conditions of bail, such as the requirement to reside at a hospital, can result in the defendant being remanded into custody.

LEGAL CONCEPTS

Not guilty by reason of insanity and Unfit to plead

The Criminal Procedure (Insanity and Unfitness to Plead Act) 1991 lays down the processes for establishing these conditions. They are defined not in the Act but from legal precedent. *Insanity* is defined according the McNaghton Rules:

> [that] at the time of committing the act the accused party was labouring under such a defect of reason, from disease of the mind, as not to know the nature and quality of the act he was doing or, if he did know it, that he did not know that what he was doing was wrong.

To be *fit to plead* a defendant should be able to:
- Understand the charge
- Understand the difference between pleading guilty and pleading not guilty
- Instruct his counsel
- Follow the evidence given in court
- Challenge a juror.

For a finding of unfitness to plead or not guilty by reason of insanity, the court must consider the evidence of two doctors, one of whom is 'approved'. If a person is found unfit to plead, then another jury is sworn in, and a 'trial of the facts' takes place to ascertain if the defendant 'did the act or made the omission charged against him'. Should this be found then 'findings are recorded that the accused is under disability and did the act or made the omission charged against him'. A finding of not guilty by reason of insanity is called a 'special verdict'. In either case, the court has four options:
- Hospital order with or without Home Office restrictions
- Guardianship order as defined by the Mental Health Act 1983
- Supervision and treatment order
- Order for absolute discharge.

Diminished responsibility

This can only be used as a defence where the offence is one of homicide. It is defined in the Homicide Act 1957 as:

> such abnormality of mind (whether arising from a condition of arrested or retarded development of mind or any inherent causes or induced by disease or injury) as substantially impaired his mental responsibility for his acts in doing or being a party to the killing.

If such a plea is successful, the conviction becomes one of manslaughter, which allows the judge wide discretion in sentencing.

Mental capacity

Mental capacity is another legal concept that is defined by precedent and has been the subject of much legal and medical discussion in the last decade. At the time of writing, there is no Act defining mental incapacity and, although the subject was considered in the Mental Health Act Code of Practice (1999), it is not formalized in the Mental Health Act 1983. Nonetheless, all doctors are likely to have to consider the issue of whether their patients have the mental capacity to take treatment decisions. There is no clearcut way of doing this but some means of proceeding is required when a patient refuses treatment advised by their doctor. This creates a conflict between the duty of care of the doctor and the patient's right of self-determination.

In determining mental capacity some basic factors need to be taken into account:

- The patient should be presumed to have capacity unless it can be shown that they have not
- The degree of mental capacity required depends on the nature of the decision, more serious decisions requiring a higher level of capacity
- If the patient has mental capacity the doctor will be acting unlawfully if s/he gives a patient a treatment without their consent, even if the patient would suffer if not given it
- What matters is the patient's mental capacity at the time of the decision, not at the time of the treatment, so a properly made 'advance directive' to refuse treatment should be respected
- If a patient does not have the requisite mental capacity, the doctor should act in the patient's 'best interests'

The case of *In re C* provided the most widely quoted criteria for deciding if a patient has capacity. These are that the patient has the capacity to:

- take in and retain treatment information
- believe it and
- weigh that information, balancing risks and needs.

In cases of doubt, a doctor should consult colleagues for advice or a second opinion and discuss the case with his/her defence organization.

COURT DIVERSION

Mentally disordered offenders have multiple disabilities that challenge community services. These offenders usually fall between services and are not regarded as an attractive or rewarding group to work with. They often have personality disorders, violence is a potential problem, substance misuse is common and the instability associated with life in and out of prison and crime usually involves periods of homelessness. Some patients do not fall within the remit of forensic psychiatric services as they may not have committed a serious offence and may not always have easily identifiable symptoms of mental illness.

What happened before court diversion?

People who are a threat to the public, likely not to attend court or homeless were usually remanded to prison while reports are compiled. This may not be the best way of obtaining reports in a disadvantaged group. The problems are that: while awaiting a psychiatric assessment in prison, there is a risk that the person may commit suicide as a direct result of mental illness; there are often delays in obtaining psychiatric assessments; and multidisciplinary assessment and treatment is not possible in a prison setting. Even when individuals were identified as ill there were delays before transfer to hospital: the person usually had to wait for a court appearance; there might not be a hospital bed available for the remanded prisoner; and a bed with the right level of security might not be available (open ward, locked ward, regional secure unit, special hospital).

If an individual was not sectionable but did suffer from a mental illness, when they attended court they were sentenced or released without any aftercare. The emphasis has up to now been on those who are deemed to require hospital admission. Similarly, there are people who are not sectionable but have unmet social-care needs that adversely influence their mental state.

Court diversion schemes

The Department of Health Circular 66/90 sought to promote diversion and discontinuance mechanisms as a means of ensuring that mentally ill offenders do not get caught up needlessly in the criminal justice system. Court diversion schemes form the main mechanism by which this philosophy has been instituted. Schemes across the UK vary in their structure, manpower requirements, level of training of individuals and number of sessions for which they are available. Most schemes include the availability of section-12-approved doctors and nurse specialists with experience of forensic psychiatry. Approved social workers, probation officers, psychologists and ward nurses are less often part of the team, but some schemes exist where their valuable contribution is incorporated.

The information collated by the court diversion scheme staff member (psychiatrist or nurse) is presented in court, along with any section papers and information about bed availability.[1] The Royal College of Psychiatrists has published guidelines for the aftercare of potentially violent or vulnerable patients discharged from inpatient psychiatric treatment.[2] The Reed report[3] suggests that similar procedures should be invoked in the case of mentally disordered offenders. Thus patients discharged from prison or hospital who have offending histories and a mental illness should be the subject of multidisciplinary discharge planning meetings.

ESSENTIAL INFORMATION

- Defendant's account of the offence
- Previous psychiatric and forensic history
- Mental state examination specifically addressing whether the mental state warrants detention in hospital, and the relationship between the offence, mental state findings at assessment and mental state findings at the time of the offence (these are usually inferred from depositions and witness reports)
- Presence of mental disorder as defined by the Mental Health Act (usually leads to section 35 or 37)

- Defendant's insight into their offending behaviour and illness
- Need for treatment and the most appropriate setting
- Dangerousness of defendant and risk of absconding

Current problems

There will always be people remanded into custody because of their offending history or because of the seriousness of their offence. Some people will develop signs of mental illness when in prison, under the stress of being in prison or because of intoxication by or withdrawal from illicit substances. Prison-based diversion schemes are being evaluated. Visiting psychiatrists still do most of the psychiatric assessments, in partnership with prison medical officers. Many schemes have no consistent source of funding. Health authorities may not wish to take on a resource-hungry patient with little added finance, even although that might mean fewer prison visits by psychiatrists and money saved by the prison service because of fewer and presumably shorter remands. There are practical problems, such as arranging transport from court to prison. There is a persistent shortage of beds to receive patients from court and prisons once they are diverted. In some instances individuals have to wait on remand while a bed is found.

REPORT WRITING

Forensic psychiatrists are often asked to write reports to assist the courts in criminal or civil matters but all psychiatrists should be able to write court reports should the need arise. Writing high-quality reports is a matter of understanding the needs of the court and practice, and the following is only a brief outline, with some essential points.

- **A report should typically consist of:**
  - An **introduction**, detailing who has requested the report and why, basic details of the nature of the case, sources of information for the report, including dates and times of interviews with the patient, and a statement that the patient has understood the purpose of the interview and has consented to the preparation of a report
  - **The body of the report**, covering the psychiatric history of the patient. This will usually follow the normal structure of a psychiatric history, including previous convictions and details of the current case from the records and from the patient's point of view. This section should cover the facts necessary to support the conclusions. Sources of information, such as interviews with relatives or from other documents, should be clearly identified
  - **Conclusions and opinion**: it is usually convenient to number the conclusions and to word these clearly using language that would be understandable to someone who is not a psychiatrist

General issues in report writing

- Make sure you understand the question the court wishes to address
- Avoid jargon and explain medical terms and drugs
- In making conclusions ensure that your opinion reflects those matters which a psychiatrist can be reasonably expected to be able to express an expert opinion, and does not deal with matters which are clearly legal and not medical
- The report should be dated and signed and the writers qualifications clearly stated on the report, including if they are approved under s12 of the Mental Health Act

Risk assessment

Risk assessment is not an exact science, and even high-quality risk management cannot eliminate the possibility of adverse incidents. Although risk assessment rating scales are becoming popular, what follows is a structure for clinical risk assessment that the author has found useful and that directs the attention of the clinician towards those factors that might be influenced by clinical behaviour.

- **Behaviours of concern**: a list of those behaviours that the patient may engage in, towards which risk management can be addressed, such as attacking a spouse, self-harm or perpetrating a robbery
- **Risk-increasing factors**: including the presence of symptoms of mental illness, drug or alcohol abuse, a poor attitude to violence or lack of insight into mental illness and the need to comply with management
- **Risk-reducing factors**: including positive factors and important negatives that reduce risk, such as a history of help-seeking behaviour and a clear relapse pattern
- **Early warning signs**: a list of factors such as sleep disturbance or poor self-care that might imply early relapse in that patient
- **Scenarios of increasing risk**: a brief description of the pattern of relapse, including time scales for the various stages
- **Risk management**: a list of suggested strategies for minimizing the impact of risk-increasing factors and maximizing the benefit of risk-reducing factors, and interventions to arrest the development of a scenario of increasing risk

FURTHER READING

British Medical Association. Assessment of mental capacity – guidance for doctors and lawyers. London: BMA, 1995. *Essential background to the issue of mental capacity.*

Chiswick D, Cope R. Practical forensic psychiatry. London: Royal College of Psychiatrists, 1995. *A good introduction to the practice of forensic psychiatry.*

Gunn J, Taylor P, ed. Forensic psychiatry – clinical, legal and ethical issues. Oxford: Butterworth Heinemann, 1993. *A good reference on all aspects of forensic psychiatry.*

Mental Health Act 1983. London: HMSO, 1983.

Mental Health Act – code of practice. London: The Stationery Office, March 1999.

In re C [1994] 1 FLR 31.

RAPE

DEFINITION

> Vaginal penetration of a woman or anal penetration of a person of either sex, against their will, without their consent or without regard to obtaining their consent.

Although rape is usually a heterosexual act (other than in institutions such as prisons), male homosexual rape is being reported more often in the UK, with several recent cases receiving widespread publicity. In the UK, women remain the more common victims. Yet there is evidence from the USA that male rape accounts for up to 10% of reported cases. Among women, in one-third of cases rape is committed by someone familiar to the victim. One-fifth of rape victims are gang-raped. Rapists are rarely mentally ill and are usually young men with little sexual experience, personality disorders, previous convictions or other antisocial behaviour. Rape is more commonly carried out by young men (over half of assailants are under 25) and over two-thirds are unskilled workers or unemployed. Younger victims are common, especially in gang-rape, where teenage victims are not uncommon. Violence accompanies rape in 80% of cases, occurring more often with older women and in gangs. A weapon may have been used to threaten the victim into submission. Although rape usually refers to vaginal intercourse, other sexual acts, often humiliating ones such as anal sex, fellatio, fondling, defecation and urination, may be involved.[4]

- **MEANINGS OF SEXUAL ASSAULT**
  - Power and control
  - Expression of aggression and hate
  - Male bravado in group rape
  - The sexual experience

- **REACTIONS IN THE VICTIM**
  - Immediate severe fear of threat to life
  - Depersonalization
  - Adjustment reactions: anxiety, depression – accompanied by intense shame and guilt, suicidal thoughts, self-harm, or self-mutilation, anger and alcohol or substance misuse
  - Post-traumatic stress disorder
  - Marital/relationship difficulties
  - Sexual dysfunction
  - Loss of job and income

MANAGEMENT

Provide a quiet comfortable room with a female member of staff. Tolerate anger and disorganized behaviour; allow time to express feelings; ensure any examination of injuries is carried out by an appropriately trained female gynaecologist with specialist forensic knowledge. Involve the police after full discussion (at victim's pace) and once the acute distress has settled. A police surgeon could carry out a detailed interview and also the physical examination if necessary. Discourage bathing until all specimens have been collected. Acute psychiatric states or severe distress may necessitate admission or short-term sedative medication. Contact with a trusted friend, 'rape crisis' organizations and ongoing support and psychotherapy should be encouraged; alternative temporary accommodation is sometimes desirable, hence social needs should be thoroughly assessed.

CHILD SEXUAL ABUSE

DEFINITION

> The involvement of dependent, developmentally immature children and adolescents in sexual activities they do not truly comprehend, to which they are unable to give informed consent; or which violate social taboos or family roles.[4] (See p. 197 for fuller account.)

The acts of abuse can involve sexual gratification by exposing children to watching sexual acts or involving them in an act. Reports to date include oral, anal and genital intercourse, and rape. Ritualistic and sadistic practices have been described. The incidence and prevalence data are not reliable, although some studies indicate that 10% of the adult population admit to sexually abusive experiences as children. The younger the child the less likely they are to be able to verbalize their experience and the more likely it is that a change in behaviour will be the main indication. If family members are involved or threats have been made, feelings of shame and guilt and a fear of damaging others may delay disclosure.

DISCLOSURE TRIGGERS

- Child's report
- Changes in behaviour
- Physical symptoms (vaginal sores, discharge, bleeding, anal bleeding and perineal tears) and injuries
- Sexually precocious behaviour and play inconsistent with the child's age; sexual preoccupations
- Allegation by parent, family member, school teacher, doctor
- Change in performance at school
- Depression
- Severe anxiety symptoms
- Acting out, deliberate self-harm, suicidality
- Anorexia
- Drug and alcohol misuse
- Prostitution

RISK FACTORS

- Parents or carers have had abusive experiences

- Previous abusive experience
- Other types of abuse (emotional, non-accidental injury)
- Parental discord, including sexual and marital difficulties
- Alcohol or drug misuse by parent or carer
- Perpetrator has a history of paedophiliac or sexual offences

ASSESSMENT

Assessment should involve an experienced child-health professional. The psychiatrist's role (if they have first contact or suspicions) is in assessing risk factors, parental mental state, family dynamics, child's developmental state, alerting child health (paediatric and/or child psychiatric) and social services that a joint assessment is necessary. Joint assessments, some of which can take place within child and adolescent services, include an assessment of parenting and child-rearing skills, problem-solving within the family and discovering and communicating the wishes of the child. This may be done indirectly through art or other forms of therapy. Child psychologists and psychotherapists have a role to play in understanding the distress, their experience and the child's wishes. Hurried intervention should be avoided as it may cause more harm. It is rare for a child to be removed from parents in an emergency. This may happen if the child discloses who the perpetrator is and a return home would expose the child to further abuse or maltreatment, or if there is severe emotional and physical damage. For an overview of the management and the essential contents of a medical report, see reference 5.

NEUROIMAGING AND PSYCHIATRY

Neuroimaging involves obtaining either a structural image of the brain, using CT or MRI, or a functional image of the brain, which involves assessing one aspect of its function. Techniques used to obtain functional images include positron emission tomography (PET), single photon emission tomography (SPET), EEG, magnetic resonance spectroscopy (MRS) and functional MRI (fMRI).

STRUCTURAL IMAGING

Magnetic resonance imaging has largely superseded CT, since it is increasingly available and gives better definition of the brain. CT involves exposure to radiation and is therefore limited as a research tool. However, because CT is widely available and cheaper than MRI, it is still often used in clinical practice.

Indications for a structural scan include:

- History of head injury or neurological disease
- Presence of neurological signs of unknown cause
- Acute confusion or gradual cognitive decline
- Dementia

- First psychosis or major personality change over the age of 50 years
- Monitoring of progression of chronic disorders
- Diagnosis of organic brain disorders.

Computerized tomography

Computerized tomography is superior to MRI in detecting bony abnormalities or calcified deposits. However, structures almost encased in bone, such as the cerebellum, are poorly visualized. CT can also be used for detection of neoplasms, infarcts, inflammation and hydrocephalus.

Magnetic resonance imaging

Magnetic resonance imaging relies on the electromagnetic energy emitted from interaction between hydrogen atoms and an external magnetic field. The most common isotope is hydrogen-1, which is a spinning proton that generates its own magnetic field. The direction of this field is random, hence the net magnetization is zero. However, when an external magnetic field is present such protons will align with the magnetic field. In addition, the protons 'precess', i.e. act like spinning tops. In MRI, applications of short-radiofrequency pulses result in all protons precessing at the same frequency and in the same direction. When the external magnetic field is switched off, energy is released by these protons as they relax to their previous state. This energy is measured to produce an image. The amount of energy released will be proportional to the density of protons in that tissue, resulting in an ability to differentiate between different tissues because of the difference in their hydrogen content.

The terms T1 and T2 refer to the relaxation times of the protons back to their original random precession. The time taken to go back to original orientation, i.e. longitudinal magnetization, is called T1 and the time taken to reduce the induced orientation, i.e. transverse magnetization, is called T2 (T1 > T2). Fluids are darker than solids in a T1-weighted image; since grey matter has more fluid in it than white matter, grey matter appears darker than white matter and cerebrospinal fluid (CSF) is dark. A T1-weighted image looks 'anatomical'. CSF in a T2-weighted image appears white.

The resolution of MRI is around 1 mm.

Compared to CT, MRI is better at differentiating white and grey matter and at visualizing the posterior fossa; axial, sagittal and coronal images can be acquired, allowing volumetric analysis. As a research tool, since there is no ionizing radiation, multiple studies are possible.

Although MRI is more expensive than CT, better discrimination of tissues can be obtained by applying different magnetic fields. The contents of the posterior fossa can be better visualized, as can parts of the temporal lobe near bone. White-matter lesions are more easily seen and MRI is now used as a gold standard for diagnosis of multiple sclerosis. Bone is not well imaged, since it contains little water. Importantly, MRI can image in any plane, allowing volumetric measurements, which are not possible with CT.

However, for obvious reasons, patients with any metal in their body – such as pacemakers or aneurysm clips – cannot have an MRI scan. Other metal implants, such as those in limbs, may not be an absolute contraindications to MRI: it depends which part of the body is to be imaged. Unless MRI is absolutely clinically indicated, pregnancy is also a contraindication. It should be noted that undergoing MRI is somewhat claustrophobic and many patients are unable to tolerate it.

FUNCTIONAL IMAGING

Functional imaging currently has little role in the diagnosis of neuropsychiatric disorders. The different techniques are used primarily as research tools. However, the situation is likely to change in the future, and the techniques will assume a more clinical role. Both PET and SPET involve use of radioactive tracers, while functional MRI and MRS use magnetic resonance imaging. PET, SPET and fMRI can be used to assess functional activity of brain tissue by assessing blood flow, metabolism or brain perfusion. fMRI also assesses blood flow by measuring the 'magnetic' difference in oxygenated and deoxygenated haemoglobin. PET and SPET can also be used to measure levels of receptors, reuptake sites or turnover of neurotransmitters, depending on the radioactive tracers that are available. Currently, fMRI is unable to do this. MRS primarily detects neuronal markers such as *N*-acetyl aspartate, creatine and phosphocreatine, and choline.

Positron emission tomography

The radioactive tracers used involve isotopes of biological elements, such as oxygen-15, carbon-11, fluorine-18. The half-life of these radioisotopes is short (^{15}O: 2 min, ^{11}C: 20 min, ^{18}F: 110 min). Therefore, production of these compounds requires an on-site cyclotron, which restricts the use of PET and increases its cost. Positrons are emitted from the isotope and travel 1–2 mm. At this point each positron combines with an electron and two gamma-photons are released, which move out at 180° to one another. Thus, from gamma rays detected simultaneously by cameras placed opposite each other around the head, the site of the radioactive tracer can be determined. Various reconstruction algorithms are used to take account of such things as attenuation, to produce tomographic images. Computerized systems can thus generate maps of where receptors, metabolism or blood flow occur in the brain. The resolution of PET is around 4–6 mm.

Positron emission tomography assesses regional cerebral blood flow after injection of $^{15}H_2O$, or regional cerebral glucose metabolism after injection of ^{18}F-deoxyglucose. Carbon-11 is commonly used to label tracers for neurotransmitter reuptake sites or receptors, such as ^{11}C-raclopride for D_2 receptors and ^{11}C-flumazenil for the γ-aminobutyric acid (GABA) benzodiazepine receptor. Fluorine-18 can also be used, in such compounds as ^{18}F-dopa to assess dopamine turnover.

The use of PET to assess cerebral blood flow has been a mainstay of research into the cognitive and motor functions of the brain. In these procedures, since

$^{15}H_2O$ has a half-life of 2 min, repeated short scans are performed with differing challenges such as motor or cognitive tasks. For instance, in a series of scans subjects might be asked to undertake a memory or verbal fluency task. The picture of blood flow during baseline is then subtracted from the blood flow during the task to get an accurate picture of blood flow associated with the task. The use of PET has been increasingly replaced by fMRI, although there are still some experiments that are better performed using PET. The disadvantage of PET in comparison to fMRI is that it involves administration of radioactivity, which is increasingly tightly controlled.

Single photon emission tomography

Single photon emission tomography is very similar to PET in that it involves the injection of a radiolabelled tracer. The radioisotopes used in SPET are technetium-99 (^{99}Tc), or radioactive iodine-123 (^{123}I), with half-lives of 6 and 13 hours respectively. These compounds are made commercially and are shipped to where the scanner is available. This reduces the cost of production. Moreover, SPET cameras are more widely available than PET cameras. Gamma rays or photons are again emitted by the radioisotopes, although these are of lower energy and do not strike the detectors coincidentally. It is therefore harder to determine their origin. Thus, resolution and sensitivity are generally less than in PET: the resolution of SPET is at best 6–7 mm and is more commonly around 11 mm. The perfusion marker of blood flow is ^{99m}Tc-HMPAO. Like PET, there are a number of tracers available for markers of neurotransmitter function such as the D_2 receptor (^{123}I-IBZM) or GABA benzodiazepine receptor (^{123}I-iomazenil).

Since it is more widely available, SPET potentially has greater clinical use than PET. One indication would be evidence of cognitive impairment in the presence of a normal structural scan. It is possible for areas to be grossly underperfused, which would show up as a deficit with ^{99m}Tc-HMPAO.

ELECTROENCEPHALOGRAPHY

The electroencephalogram is a recording of the electric potential generated by both inhibitory and excitatory discharges from neurones. Since the electrodes are placed on the scalp, the electrical activity recorded is only representative of the activity at the cortical surface. Generally, the EEG involves minimal discomfort to the patient and can be performed either while lying in a clinic or while walking around. In order to gain activity from the inferior temporal lobe, sphenoidal electrodes may be used. Such an EEG is generally performed as part of the workup prior to incision of part of the temporal lobe for refractory epilepsy.

The recordings for EEGs detect alterations in cortical activity by measuring differences in voltage (10–100 μV) or frequency (0.5–40 Hz). There are four normal EEG frequencies, delta rhythm (0.1–3.9 Hz), theta rhythm (4.1–7.9 Hz), alpha rhythm (8–13 Hz) and beta rhythm (13–14 Hz). The normal awake EEG is predominantly alpha rhythm, which is maximal in the occipital region. The alpha rhythm attenuates when the eyes are open or when engaged in cognitive tasks such as mental arithmetic. The alpha rhythm is also more pronounced on the non-dominant hemisphere and alteration in this pattern may result from underlying neuropathology. The beta rhythm predominates in the frontocentral regions and replaces the alpha rhythm during mental activity. As the person becomes relaxed and sedated the beta activity becomes more prominent. Delta activity is normally only seen in very young children, and during sleep in adults.

The EEG undergoes changes during life. Both delta and beta rhythms are prominent in young children but alpha rhythm replaces them in the frontal region, the temporal and parietal region and lastly in the occipital region after the age of 5 years. The adult pattern is reached in late adolescence. In some people frontal theta and posterior temporal delta waves may persist; this is referred to as an immature EEG and is associated with personality disorder. The last change in rhythm occurs around the seventh decade, when delta rhythms make a reappearance and alpha rhythms reduce in voltage and frequency.

Other patterns that may be seen in normal EEGs include lambda waves, mu waves and K complexes. Lambda waves are seen in the occipital region and reflect eye movements. Mu waves replace the alpha rhythm in the motor cortex and are reduced by contralateral limb movement. K complexes are brief bursts of high-voltage slow waves that may emerge during non-REM (rapid eye movement) sleep.

By contrast, spikes and waves are abnormal constituents of the EEG. Spikes are high peak discharges that rise and fall rapidly, while waves rise rapidly but fall more slowly. Spikes alternating with delta waves are known as wave and spike 'discharges' and these occurring at a rhythm of 3 Hz are a classic reflection of simple absence epilepsy. Creutzfeldt–Jakob disease is associated with repeated generalized irregular spike and slow-wave complexes.

Activation procedures may also be used during the recording of the EEG, either to bring out activity normally hidden during wakefulness or to clarify suspected abnormal patterns such as occur in epilepsy. Hyperventilation is used to increase the excitability of cortical cells secondary to the hypocapnic vasoconstriction. Photic stimulation (lights flashed at between 8 and 15 Hz) should result in the occipital alpha rhythm adjusting to the same rate. This technique is also used to bring out epileptic foci. Drugs such as barbiturates or neuroleptics may also be used to do this.

Most psychotropic drugs affect the EEG. Benzodiazepines and barbiturates increase beta and delta rhythms while reducing alpha rhythms. Tricyclic antidepressants increase delta and beta rhythms. Depressants increase delta and beta rhythms. Similarly, antipsychotics at lower doses increase beta rhythms and at higher doses increase delta and beta rhythms. Lithium only induces changes at toxic levels, by increasing delta or beta rhythms. Somewhat paradoxically, as described above barbiturates, benzodiazepines and antipsychotics can be used to enhance epileptic activity.

Electroconvulsive therapy can result in changes in the EEG for a period of months after a course of treatment. The alpha rhythm may disappear completely and be replaced with slower waves such as beta and delta rhythms.

Electroencephalography does have some limitations. A normal EEG may be present with people with neuropathology and up to 20% of adults may have an abnormal EEG pattern. Although it gives good temporal information, its special localization is a relative disadvantage compared to newer neuroimaging techniques. EEG can never be used on its own to diagnose any disorder but is useful in providing more information. It is most commonly used to investigate sleep disorders and epilepsy.

Sleep

As a person falls asleep, the beta rhythm becomes less pronounced, with the alpha rhythm becoming more apparent. Sleep is 'staged' by its EEG pattern. Stage 1 is characterized by gradual disappearance of the alpha rhythm and increasing presence of delta and theta rhythms (slower). Sharp waves may appear at the vertex. In stage 2, these slower rhythms dominate, with sleep spindles (sinusoidal 12–14 Hz of 0.5 s) and K complexes. Delta waves are uniformly present in stage 3 and sleep spindles and K complexes are not so common. By stage 4, almost all the EEG is delta waves, with no sleep spindles or K complexes.

The cycle from stage 1 through to stage 4 takes about 90 minutes and occurs up to five times per night. REM sleep is associated with an EEG appearance more like an awake EEG, but the person is deeply asleep. In addition to signs of arousal such as tachycardia, dilated pupils and increased respiration, eye movement is rapid and conjugate. Dreaming occurs during REM and if the person is awakened, recall of dreams is more likely than if awakened in another stage of sleep. The amount of REM time decreases with age, being 50% of sleep time in childhood and only 25% in adults. REM sleep dominates in the latter half of the night. Increased REM, or REM rebound, can be seen following sleep deprivation, withdrawal of benzodiazepines, barbiturates or alcohol.

Nightmares

Nightmares occur during REM sleep and are therefore more likely in the later part of the night. They are common in childhood and rare in adults.

Night terrors

Characteristically, the child awakens terrified and may shout out but goes back to sleep with little memory of the event in the morning. These episodes occur in stages 3 and 4 of sleep and hence are more likely to happen earlier in the night than nightmares. A family history is common. Night terrors rarely persist into adulthood.

Sleepwalking

This also arises out of stages 3 and 4 of sleep and is mostly found in children. It occurs primarily in males and there is frequently a family history. Sleepwalking is an automatism and there is debate about how complex the movements can be. Although self-harm is rare, the bedroom may have to be made safer.

Narcolepsy

Narcolepsy is characterized by short periods of daytime sleep (narcoleptic attacks). The EEG shows REM. Cataplexy – sudden loss of muscle tone – may occur and result in the patient falling to the floor. Narcoleptic episodes are often triggered by strong emotional stimuli, particularly laughter. Other associated phenomena include sleep paralysis and hypnagogic hallucinations. Narcolepsy is strongly familial and is associated with the human lymphocyte antigen DR2 (DR15/DQ6).

Treatment involves stimulants to combat daytime sleepiness, such as amfetamine-like drugs (methylphenidate, dexamfetamine, mazindol), and SSRIs to help cataplexy and hypnagogic hallucinations.

Epilepsy

Epilepsy is the occurrence of two or more seizures per year. The prevalence of people having one seizure is 2% but only 0.5% have epilepsy. Most patients suffer their first fit before the age of 18 years, with the incidence dropping throughout later life. Epilepsy can be broadly divided into *generalized epilepsy*, where there is widespread involvement, and *partial epilepsy*, where the focus is more limited. Partial seizures may develop into a generalized pattern. Partial epilepsy is more common than generalized. Generalized epilepsy includes *tonic–clonic*, *absence* and *atonic* seizures, while partial or focal epilepsy includes *simple (jacksonian)* or *complex* seizures, in which consciousness is preserved and lost respectively. Complex partial seizures typically arise in the temporal lobe. Absence or petit mal seizures are characterized by brief lapses of consciousness. While the cause of most epilepsy is unknown, some are genetic, drug-induced 'intoxication' or withdrawal, or secondary to head injury or tumour. There is no 'personality' associated with epilepsy.

Diagnosis

As already stated, an abnormal EEG may be present in normal individuals and the converse is also true, 20% of people with epilepsy showing a normal EEG pattern. Activation processes can be used to bring out abnormal patterns. A classical pattern of the interictal EEG is spikes and waves at alpha, theta and delta frequencies. These may be focal or generalized, synchronized or desynchronized. Absence seizures are associated with a spike and wave pattern at 3 Hz. Tonic–clonic seizures are also associated with spike and wave complexes but at a higher frequency.

Diagnosis of epilepsy relies primarily on a comprehensive history. Investigations often play a lesser role. Psychiatrists become involved in the care of people with epilepsy because of the reported higher incidence in epilepsy of psychiatric disorders, such as depression, suicide and neuroses. At times, the symptom of aura can be mistaken for a psychiatric illness. In treating psychiatric illness in a patient with epilepsy, caution is required. As mentioned, many psychotropic drugs can affect the EEG and the seizure threshold is generally reduced. In addition, many antiepileptic drugs cause depression.

Syndromes associated with epilepsy

Some patients describe a prodrome, which usually lasts for days and includes affective changes, insomnia, headache and irritability. In patients with complex partial epilepsy arising from the temporal lobe, auras are often present. The patient can describe feelings of depersonalization, derealization, fear, anxiety or depression. Usually these last for a few seconds before the rest of the seizure supervenes. It is these phenomena that can be mistaken for a psychiatric illness.

After an epileptic fit, automatisms may occur. These are brief periods of usually simple behaviours such as lip-smacking or hand movements in clouded consciousness. Less frequently, automatisms can involve complex behaviours. Patients have no recall of this period. Twilight states also occur post-ictally and involve the experience of intense hallucinations.

Psychiatric syndromes are more common in patients with complex partial seizures, most of which involve the temporal lobe. Temporal lobe epilepsy is associated with a schizophreniform psychosis. There is a two- to threefold greater risk of psychosis. Differences between this concession and schizophrenia include preservation of affective reactivity, no family history of psychosis, normal premorbid personality and an illness that generally begins at least 10 years after the onset of epilepsy. Psychotic symptoms usually worsen with increasing seizure frequency but, more rarely, 'forced normalization' may be seen in which, during periods of seizures, the psychosis resolves. Personality disorders are also more prevalent in people with epilepsy, most commonly borderline.

Episodic dyscontrol syndrome is associated with unprovoked violence and with an abnormal EEG. It is a contentious diagnosis.

Non-epileptic seizures

Distinguishing between seizures and non-epileptic or pseudoseizures can be very difficult. In some instances they coexist. Pseudoseizures occur more commonly in women and usually involve unresponsiveness and movements that do not fit into any known seizure pattern. Gradual onset and longer duration are clues that seizures are non-epileptic. They often occur in the presence of others and respond poorly to anticonvulsant medication. EEG telemetry (continuous recording) can be used to aid diagnosis. A normal EEG is observed and no rise in prolactin levels is seen. Pseudoseizures can be considered to be a type of conversion disorder and managed using similar strategies.

THE SKIN AND PSYCHIATRY

PRE-EXISTING SKIN CONDITION

Up to 80% of patients attending a dermatologist have a psychiatric disorder. The social and physical distress caused to patients by a pre-existing skin condition and its comprehensive management may lead to the development of low self-esteem, anxiety and depressive disorders. This is particularly evident among teenagers with acne but of course those with severe psoriasis and eczema usually have to devote much of their daily lives to managing their skin. Unsightly blemishes or eruptions on highly visible areas (hands, face, upper body, genitals) encourage social withdrawal and isolation. Our outward appearance influences the way people react to us socially and hence shapes our sense of self and identity. A change of appearance or a chronic and severely disabling skin condition is experienced as a loss event and parallels can be drawn with bereavement. The daily rituals necessary for some (tar baths, creams, etc.) will occupy them to the exclusion of a job or active social life.

Support groups are helpful but, should significant depressive and anxiety symptoms develop, more focused counselling and cognitive behavioural psychotherapy will be required. If biological symptoms of depression arise or the symptoms are severely disabling, pharmacological treatments should be considered, although their adverse effects could mean that they are unsuitable.

Pre-existing conditions may deteriorate for several reasons. Severe depressive symptoms could prevent patients from caring for their skin adequately; this includes using creams and baths, attending for assessment and maintaining hygiene. Anxiety disorders may be accompanied by excessive scratching, preventing healing and also damaging the skin further by lichenification. Scratching may be used to relieve tension or overtly to inflict pain.

NO PRE-EXISTING SKIN CONDITION

Stress may itself precipitate certain skin conditions and alleviating stress is known to play a part in managing some skin conditions. Neurodermatitis, pruritus ani, eczema, psoriasis, urticaria, alopecia and rosacea are common examples. Obsessive hand-washing, or taking bleach baths for obsessive cleanliness are examples of behaviour that will not only exacerbate skin conditions but also precipitate them. Skin conditions often accompany ulcerative colitis and rheumatoid arthritis, each of which has recognized emotional associations.

Patients suffering from self-mutilation and deliberate self-harm will have unsightly scars and may require cosmetic surgery, especially if the damage was done to socially exposed skin areas and the patient has recovered and wants a normal lifestyle.

Factitious disorders such as dermatitis artefacta require careful unravelling of the motivation that underlies the behaviour. Seeking the illness role, desire for care and love, avoiding other immediate conflicts, deep-seated aggressive personality traits and a sense of injustice may motivate some. Repeated wound breakdown or atypical wounds and healing patterns should alert the clinician.

PSYCHIATRIC DISORDER AND PREOCCUPATION WITH SKIN

Dermatological delusions about infestation, parasitosis and deformity are very difficult to treat unless they are part of a major depressive syndrome. Monosymptomatic delusions, although uncommon, present significant problems of management. Pimozide has traditionally been prescribed but is less often used now because of its potential adverse myocardial effects. Antidepressants and cognitive behavioural strategies are worth pursuing. Such delusions can arise in schizophrenia, paranoid states, organic brain states and alcohol and drug withdrawal. Bizarre reasoning may lead to self-mutilation.

Dysmorphophobia involves an excessive preoccupation with a feature (nose shape, skin blemish, etc.) where there is no apparent abnormality. The most common areas presented are the scalp, face and genital area. Depression and comorbid disorders should be excluded (e.g. social problems, sexually transmitted disease, marital or sexual problems as well as dementia, paranoid psychosis, schizophrenia and visual sensory impairment).

COMORBID PSYCHIATRIC AND SKIN CONDITIONS

Psychotropic drugs can cause skin eruptions. Most commonly, lithium treatment can exacerbate pre-existing psoriasis. Light-sensitive dermatitis is common in patients on neuroleptics (especially chlorpromazine) and a sun screen should be advised.

BURNS

These present unique problems. Burns may arise from attempts at self-harm, accidental injury or abusive and assaultative experiences. The psychopathology needing attention will reflect these diverse possibilities. Common to all of these will be bereavement (accompanying disfigurement), disability and depression because of limitations of activity and rehabilitation required if the burns are severe. Self-harm attempts will require simultaneous psychiatric assessment and treatment; traumatic assaultative and abusive experiences will require specialist psychological treatments specific to these problems.

COMMON STRATEGIES

- Specialist support groups exist for most common skin conditions
- Identify comorbid psychopathology and treat at the same time
- Psychological and pharmacological treatments are necessary for specific disorders such as schizophrenia and major depression
- Long-term support and psychotherapy are necessary adjuncts to rehabilitation where the level of disability is severe
- Rationalize the drug regimen
- Consider social care needs for independent living

IMPROVING TREATMENT ADHERENCE

The antipsychotic effects of neuroleptics were established in the early 1950s. The effectiveness of prophylactic treatment was established later, in the 1970s. Up to 60% of those who stop taking their medication relapse, compared with about 16% of those who persist. Studies examining the relapse rates among patients who stop taking medication indicate that as many as 80% suffer a relapse.

Rates of non-compliance with antipsychotic medication range from 11% to 80%. Almost half of patients are reported to be non-compliant within the first year of treatment and over two-thirds within the first 2 years. It is estimated that almost one-fifth of psychiatric inpatients do not take their drugs regularly, despite close supervision.

The word 'compliance' reflects an unequal power relationship and allocates blame for a failure of treatment to the patient. The basis of most psychoeducational programmes is that collaboration rather than a demand for compliance will improve the chances of adherence to treatment regimens. It is established that a failure to take medication does not account for all those who relapse. Family factors (expressed emotion), social stressors, life events, illness and cultural factors also affect the likelihood of relapse.

STRATEGIES TO IMPROVE EFFECTIVENESS OF DRUG TREATMENT

- **Overview of current information: written and verbal**
- **Teach participants about symptoms, and the effects and side-effects of medication**
- **Increase participants' awareness of environmental stress and its relationship to relapse**
- **Prepare patients and relatives for early warning signs of relapse**
- **Identify individual strengths and weaknesses and teach coping strategies**
- **Increase collaboration between the patients, their families and staff**
- **Prepare participants for discharge to enable them to cope on their own**
- **Encourage networking among families to lessen isolation and stigma**
- **Empower patients to take a greater role in their own treatment**
- **Arrange self-administration of medication and evaluation of its effect**
- **Keep the regimen simple**
- **Tailor to daily rituals**
- **Provide explicit written instructions**
- **Implement changes to drug regimens gradually**
- **Involve the patient in the decision-making process**
- **Provide warm, positive feedback for compliance and attainment of the therapeutic goals**
- **Schedule appointments before patients are discharged**
- **Shorten the waiting period for appointments**
- **Use prompts to encourage patients to keep their appointments**

- **Take an interest in, and have concern about, compliance**
- **Ensure that the patient and all significant contacts are well informed about medication**
- **Enlist the help of the patient's family in improving compliance**
- **Use the minimum amount of medication possible and monitor adverse effects**
- **Consider alternative regimens using medication with fewer side-effects (clozapine, risperidone)**

Substance-misusing patients may require higher neuroleptic doses; disorganized living style adds to uncertainty about timing of medication, as does short-term memory impairment after acute intoxication. Those with physical disabilities or those who live far away from the clinic may find it too difficult to attend reviews. Educational interventions that involve the family, daily rituals and regular contact with a health-care professional will help. Among patients with poor memories or organizing capacity, dosette boxes are invaluable, allowing patients to know when they have missed a particular dose.

PERSISTENT PSYCHOTIC SYMPTOMS: NON-PHARMACOLOGICAL STRATEGIES

A quarter to a third of patients with schizophrenia have hallucinations or delusional beliefs despite adequate doses of antipsychotic medication. Some patients show persistent and disabling negative symptoms such as apathy and social withdrawal and may still sometimes experience hallucinations or paranoia but are reluctant to disclose this or are unable to make sense of and report their experience. Trials of clozapine and risperidone are promising but some patients show a less than optimal response or refuse to try these newer drug therapies. Recent attention has focused on psychological approaches among the severely mentally ill with persistent hallucinations and delusions.[6,7]

STRATEGIES FOR PERSISTENT HALLUCINATIONS

- BEHAVIOURAL REGIMEN
  - Social reinforcement
  - Time out and token punishment
  - Assertive training to avoid frustration and aggression
- ACTIVITY
  - Exercise to improve confidence, mobility, reduce weight and improve mood symptoms
  - Posture: lying down, gentle exercise, walking
  - Leisure: painting, sewing, carpentry

- **COGNITIVE STRATEGIES**
  - Belief modification: target particular beliefs; induce cognitive dissonance about them, reality test them, offer alternative normalizing explanations
  - Thought stopping, biofeedback and self-control
- **SENSORY**
  - Wearing earplugs
  - Listening to music or watching television
  - Exposure to hallucinations: repeat content aloud; listen for fixed times in the day only
  - Arguing with voices
- **OTHERS**
  - Increasing or reducing social contact
  - Stimulus control: modulating contact with triggers or cues, especially if other urgent tasks needs completion
  - Self-instruction: anxiety management and rehearsal techniques to talk oneself away from distress
  - Some patients find temporary relief by the use of complementary treatments, which probably reduce arousal and levels of anxiety

RELIGION AND MENTAL HEALTH

Mental illness may present with statements of regret for transgressing religious norms, but more commonly there is a religious slant to the beliefs present in psychotic illness. There is evidence that things are changing: more recently, psychotic phenomena tend to be furnished with a pseudoscientific explanation, such as radio transmitters or other electronic devices. The decline of religious phenomena among delusional explanations may be related to secularization in the West, yet inevitably, when people have been exposed to religious teachings, there is always the possibility that they will deploy religious ideology to explain their experience of illness.

Religious phenomena have been linked to temporal lobe abnormalities; this is of interest as schizophrenia has, since the development of neuroimaging techniques, been linked to neurodevelopmental abnormalities of the temporal lobe. Hyper-religiosity and a preoccupation with philosophy are also described as features of the epileptoid personality type, thought to be associated with temporal lobe epilepsy. Temporal lobe damage or developmental abnormality can result in religious delusions; perhaps there is a biological basis to religious thinking.

Religious beliefs, as discussed above, are influential in the appraisal process when a person experiences illness. The conclusions such a person draws from an experience will inevitably be consistent with their religious ideology. If confession can provide an adequate means of dealing with daily anxieties and ambivalent conflicts about one's morality, then distress is allayed. The confusion surrounding a mental illness can be mitigated by the certainties of religious ritual and belief, which can give an alternative explanation of the meaning of the cosmos to the reductionist scientific viewpoint.

From the perspective of Western society, in which religious beliefs are common and beliefs in magic uncommon, patients describing 'magic' may be more readily labelled as mentally ill than those describing religious beliefs. Societies with standards of normal behaviour often specify times and conditions under which abnormal behaviour may be displayed. These 'rites of reversal' or 'symbolic inversions' usually take place at festivals or special occasions. However, such behaviours are strictly controlled, since their context and timing is arranged in advance.

In many non-Western societies, individuals experiencing interpersonal distress or conflict may display behaviours that, to a Western-trained psychiatrist, are sufficiently deviant from his/her norms to be identified as mental illness. Thus in many parts of the world people freely engage in states of possession, including hallucinatory states in which special messages are received from the ancestors or from spirits. Possession serves as a culturally sanctioned way of expressing distress, or views or wishes not consistent with the rules of society. Ecstatic states and glossolalia (speaking in tongues) may form part of some religious practice, but are not common in the West. These states may be misdiagnosed by a Western mental health professional as illness.

Thus unusual rituals or states or behaviours that are not familiar to an observer may be perfectly consistent with a different form of religious worship but appear as mental illness. Mental health professionals have always to be wary of situations in which misdiagnosis may occur. Religious beliefs can be difficult to disentangle from psychopathology if a knowledge of the patient's religious beliefs is absent. Therapists should assess and approach a religious group using its vocabulary and through the social organization of the religious group. When a possession state or glossolalia is deemed to be abnormal by those who share a culture with a patient, it is more likely to be a symptom of illness.

Religion can be used adaptively or maladaptively and can have a positive or negative impact. Sharing religion with others of the same ideology secures a supportive culture in which one feels understood and accepted. Religion is multidimensional and social support is one valuable aspect of it. Religious support systems may compete with statutory services to be the preferred option and it may be that for a particular patient they serve a more satisfactory solution; knowing that one can share in the care of others and oneself in a community can give a sense of purpose to an otherwise isolated group of people who are no longer in stable relationships or have lost their loved ones. God can be seen as a protective influence and belief in ultimate salvation can remove the intensity of anxiety surrounding a situation the outcome of which is unclear.

Religious leaders are influential and a patient's peers in a religious community may be able to persuade and support a patient in seeking help and engaging in services. Of particular value is the view of a patient's religious leader about the beliefs and behaviour in which a potential patient engages. The leader may suggest a complete absence of any abnormality or may point out what discrepancies there are with healthy religious activity, thus further improving the reliability with which diagnoses can be made across religious boundaries. If models of health and illness are shared then better understanding of a problem is possible. Where models differ (in the absence of delusional beliefs) then treatment offered may be rejected as it would break religious taboos and threaten the safety and security that religion affords to those in distress.

RELIGION AND MENTAL HEALTH: ARENAS OF SHARED INFLUENCE

- **ILLNESS EXPERIENCE AND DEALING WITH DISTRESS**
  - Ways of conceptualizing misfortune: explanations of illness experience
  - Making sense of events: a punishment or suffering sent by God that is to be accepted
  - Constructs about help-seeking
  - Prescriptions about dealing with strong emotions such as anger
- **RITES OF PASSAGE: FAMILY, MARRIAGE, CHILDREN, BIRTH AND DEATH**
  - Adhering to prescribed patterns of marriage: who, when, why and why not
  - Acceptable family structures, single parenthood
  - Ways of dealing with family disagreements, distress and social problems
  - Marriage arrangements: limitations of partner's religion, culture, social class
  - Premarital sex may be acceptable or forbidden
  - Sexual activity: frequency, prohibitions, special observances and taboos, homosexuality
  - Children: education, style of reinforcing societal norms
  - Role of women in society
  - Ceremonies for birth and death
- **RELIGIOUS PRACTICE, RITUAL, IDEOLOGY AND ORGANIZATIONS**
  - Emotional support from religious certainty leading to hope and forward planning
  - Emotional support from one's friends and religious leaders
  - Work may be seen to be an essential to fulfilment
  - Pathways to salvation: what acts must be done and in what time-frame
  - Rules by which one lives – is state law separate from religious law?
  - Definitions of deviance reinforced
  - Prayer and religious ritual: distraction, hope, communication with one's self
  - A sense of belonging

FUNCTIONS OF RELIGION

- Religion serves as a filter, articulating the illness experience in mental disorder
- Religion, metaphors and idioms of distress are used to verbalize the appraisal of illness experience

- Religious content of beliefs in mental illness
- Religion informs help-seeking
- Clinically difficulties arise when trying to differentiate between religious fervour, ecstatic states, possession and mental illness
- Religious communities may have their own coping strategies (prayer/confession) – these should be considered in the treatment plan

THE EMERGENCY CROSS-CULTURAL PSYCHIATRIC ASSESSMENT

COMMUNICATION AND CULTURAL DISTANCE

These are general guidelines aimed at ensuring safe and sensitive practice and do not represent a recipe of how to do it culture by culture. Before an assessment, note the first and preferred language in which the patient communicates. If this is not English, find an interpreter. Be aware of your own and the patient's body language. During the initial part of the assessment try to identify idioms of distress and 'emotional' words used by the patient.

PITFALLS IN THE CROSS-CULTURAL ASSESSMENT

- **Cultural camouflage**: mentally ill patients may encourage your perception of not understanding their culture and rationalize their symptoms as being in accord with their culture. Do not dismiss a patient's or relative's complaints if you are persuaded that there is enough evidence of mental illness, that the patient needs urgent treatment and that home treatment will fail
- You may be under pressure from relatives and friends not to admit or label because of stigma, impact on self-esteem and fear of being 'locked away'. If during a crisis you are unable to address all the patient's, family's and advocate's concerns, arrange a special meeting with them to convey your concerns after the patient is 'safely managed'. Make sure you convey the risks you are taking, the risks you are prepared to take and the risks they are asking you to take. Where there is doubt about the assessment and diagnosis, if all parties are prepared to share the risks and the patient is not in need of hospitalization, then more creative treatment interventions can be considered in terms of location, type of intervention and personnel involved. The more difficult the decision the more important it is that a proper case conference is held as soon as possible, involving all parties
- Be aware that delusional beliefs, religious beliefs and degree of insight are very difficult to assess conclusively in a different culture
- Terms describing ethnic identity do not convey the degree of identification with any specific community, religion or language and should be carefully applied. The limitations of such categories for each patient should be specified

- Identify during the assessment the sense of belonging, family structure, family roles, where the patient fits into these, role expectations in the context of their culture and styles of dealing with distress or conflict. Second- and third-generation children have varying degrees of Western identity, views, health beliefs and religious commitment
- Anthropology has shed much light on the limitations of Western psychiatry yet it remains a Western science in itself. Thus there is always the possibility that value judgements and culturally insensitive practice enter the interaction between patient and health professional
- Do not underestimate the impact of discrimination in the patient's life – this will undermine trust
- Do not miss culturally consistent behaviours that differ in quality or quantity from those that the patient's reference group consider to be within cultural bounds

SETTING UP THE ASSESSMENT

- Know your limits: be aware of your own culture and how your skills may therefore be blunted
- Know the patient's limits: assume nothing about the patient; assess which is the predominant group with which the patient identifies
- Know the family's limits: their language limitations, sense of urgency and crisis and capacity to support the patient should home-based treatment be chosen
- Know the interpreter's limits: meet with him/her before the assessment; ensure the interpreter is from the same culture, identify sources of difference (e.g. dialect, religion). Agree the method of working together: literal translation of all material; will you use the interpreter to assess the cultural context of complaints? Does the patient have any objections to this particular interpreter?
- Identify the most important information you need
- Identify the most important things the patient wants to find out
- Identify the most important things the patient's family and friends want to know

PRACTICE POINTS

- For each of the parties involved in the consultation elicit: first language, place of birth, religion, parental place of birth, self-defined ethnicity, identifications with specific cultural groups
- Define and redefine terms used by you and the patient to ensure a shared understanding of the problem
- Critically ask for clarification about signs or symptoms that seem unusual or simply bizarre: explore the experience, and then the meaning of the experience to the patient and their family
- Do not be judgemental about patterns of communication or domination of an interview by one family member. This may be their designated role

- Be sensitive to the effect of anything about your actions, the setting or the referral mode that jeopardizes trust. For example, communicate that total confidentiality will be observed
- Specifically, be sensitive to religious and social taboos within the patient's culture. For instance, women may prefer to be seen by a woman
- Do not ask relatives and children to interpret
- Involve independent advocates early; this should be done with the patient's agreement
- You must discuss the findings with an independent person properly familiar with the patient's cultural background. This preferably should be a member of the health professions but many voluntary organizations offer this advocacy role
- If you do not know for certain, do not assume anything about the patient
- Some patients will express explanations of their state that may sound like delusional content: for example, in one study explanatory models among Indians included sorcery (10%), possession by demons or deities (33%), humoral imbalance (15%), violations of taboo (5%) and external stressors (33%)

MANAGEMENT

- This consists of carefully balancing the treatment requirements with the patient's wishes, taking account of cultural distance and that you may be making a decision based on much less information than is usual. This makes it more likely that you will make the wrong decision and requires that you carry out a careful risk assessment. Do not prescribe symptomatically if the diagnosis is unclear. This will lead to false expectations on the part of the patient and may expose them to adverse side-effects that render them less inclined to return or take medication in the future
- If the situation is not urgent and there is insufficient time, arrange a further assessment time. This will allow you to think about the patient's presentation, obtain supervision and obtain corroborative information from past records, doctors, social workers and other family members familiar with the cultural context. Let the patient know that you will be making enquiries. They may object
- If the situation is urgent and a crisis admission is required, avoid medication if possible until further assessment on the ward has taken place. Do not admit under section in the following circumstances:
  - Linguistic isolation or the absence of an interpreter
  - Where the presentation does not make sense and further assessment would be helpful but the patient refuses admission
  - Where there are no immediate indicators of major mental illness or risk of self-harm

  If you are sure that there are major signs or symptoms of mental illness and/or a risk of serious self-harm, admit the patient. Discuss the plan with the patient and their relatives. Be aware that placing patients in an unfamiliar ward environment may exacerbate their mental state and necessitate urgent medication. Be aware that the relatives may be unable to manage the patient on their own despite their best intentions and their wish to take the patient home in accord with his/her wishes.

CULTURE-BOUND SYNDROMES

These are defined as a group of disorders confined to a single culture or area. They are popular examination topics but usually, when such exotic disorders are discovered, there is a flurry of case reports indicating the existence of a syndrome in other cultures also; the original pathological interpretation placed on a behaviour or syndrome retrospectively is identified as having arisen out of poor communication and culturally based ethnocentric value judgements by the observer.

Such syndromes have a range of symbolic meanings that are not readily translated across cultures and are often embedded in the sociopolitical history of a society. Agoraphobia, parasuicide and anorexia have been described as culture-bound syndromes of the industrialized nations.[8]

Some of the better-known culture-bound syndromes are listed.

- **Koro** was originally described in Chinese men and is a fear of the penis shrinking into the abdomen. Some men even tie a piece of string around the penis to prevent it disappearing or ask their partner to hold on to it. It is regarded as an anxiety state
- **Dhat** was originally described among Indian men, who characteristically complain of loss of semen in the urine. They have multiple aches and report that loss of semen is making them weak. It is regarded as an anxiety state but reports indicate that it does respond to antidepressant medication
- **Windigo** was originally described in North America as a compulsive desire to become a cannibal. This syndrome has since been discredited as an artefact of poor communication and premature assumptions about the behaviour
- **Susto**, also known as soul loss, is a syndrome from Latin America. It is considered to be a depressive state
- **Shinkeishitsu** is an anxiety state described among Japanese men. It is a syndrome of obsessionality and anxiety symptoms
- **Latah** consists of automatic stylized imitative behaviour, including posturing and the utterance of obscenities, immediately after a startle reaction. It seems that the biological basis of this exaggerated startle reaction is common to all cultures but it is identified and reinforced so that it has some social and cultural meaning in South East Asia

It is better not to try and shape the psychiatric presentation to one of these syndromes but rather to specify what aspects of the patient's presentation might be better understood by comparison with them, as they are likely to undergo change in any case.

POSSESSION STATES

The term 'possession' means many things to the lay public but usually evokes a picture of demonic possession. Such states are reported generally as the experience of a spirit entering and taking control of an individual. Various perspectives deriving from disciplines including sociology, anthropology, theology and psychopathology have enabled a better understanding of possession.[9] Possession states are common everywhere and are culturally accepted by about 90% of the world's population.[10]

Demonic possession is characterized by sudden sensory and motor changes (anaesthesia to pain and temperature; feats of enormous strength), sudden alteration of conscious level and an audible (to observers) change in voice. It is this type of possession in which religious ideology plays the greatest part, although the mechanism may be dissociative according to Western theories; specifically there appears to be no objective account of a change in level of consciousness. Features vary from culture to culture so that the manifestation and resolution of such states are culturally determined in accord with the lay and religious body of knowledge about such phenomena. Indeed, for exorcism to fail is regarded in some cultures as evidence of mental illness.

Sociocultural possession states are regarded as culturally sanctioned methods of resolving interpersonal and community distress where other methods of resolution do not exist. Commonly, these are cited to occur among those who have no culturally appropriate method of protesting; they are common among women, for example, in cultures where women's status is not high and where they have placed upon them impossible expectations and obligations (Zar possession states). This type of possession and its treatment are socialized events and serve a function within a society.

Finally, possession as a symptom of mental illness is usually manifest as delusional beliefs about being possessed. The illness then would not respond to exorcism.

PSYCHIATRIC DIFFERENTIAL DIAGNOSIS

- **Schizophrenia, affective disorders and schizoaffective states**
- **Brief reactive psychosis**
- **Personality disorders: multiple and borderline types**
- **Organic disorders**
- **Temporal lobe epilepsy**
- **Head injury**
- **Psychoactive substance intoxication**
- **Sensory deprivation and other extreme states of deprivation**

MANAGEMENT[9]

- Possession states require a comprehensive social, psychiatric, biological and cultural assessment. A full psychiatric history, mental state and physical examination are required. It is important to have a thorough neurological assessment because of the possibility of an organic disorder presenting in this way
  - Ritualized trance states (e.g. mediums assuming conscious control of events)
  - Suggestibility phenomena (e.g. faith healing, witchcraft, voodoo)
  - Dissociative phenomena (include brief psychosis or conversion symptoms)
  - Delusional possession as a symptom of a mental illness
- The management is the same as for the generic psychiatric disorder diagnosed; notably those with dissociative features benefit from benzodiazepines to contain symptoms (rather than neuroleptics), along with abreaction and psychotherapy aimed at identifying the conflicts. Those with delusional possession require antipsychotic pharmacological and psychotherapeutic (cognitive behavioural) treatments. Traditional culturally sanctioned mechanisms of resolving distress are likely to be unsuccessful if applied to patients who have delusional possession states but may be helpful in those with dissociative disorders
- The difficulty lies in distinguishing the dissociative group from those with suggestibility states. Therefore the assessment of suggestibility, ritualized and dissociative states will require consultation with those having expert knowledge about religious, cultural, spiritual and sociological aspects of possession states. Members of the community to which the patient belongs should be consulted at all stages of the assessment and treatment process

REFERENCES

1. Carson, D. Doctors in the witness box. Br J Hosp Med 1985; 33, 283–286.
2. Royal College of Psychiatrists. Good medical practice in the aftercare of potentially violent or vulnerable patients discharged from inpatient psychiatric treatment. London: Royal College of Psychiatrists, 1991.
3. Reed, J. Review of the health and social services for mentally disordered offenders and others requiring similar services. Final Summary Report. London: HMSO, 1992.
4. Bancroft J. Human sexuality and its problems. Edinburgh: Churchill Livingstone, 1989.
5. DHSS. Diagnosis of child sexual abuse: guidance for doctors. London: HMSO, 1988.
6. Kingdon D, Turkington D. Cognitive behaviour therapy of schizophrenia. New York: Guilford Press, 1994.
7. Huckle PL, Palia SS. Managing resistant schizophrenia. Br J Hosp Med 1993; 50: 467–471.

8. Helman CG. Culture, health and illness. Oxford: Butterworth Heinemann, 1990.
9. Perera S, Bhui K, Dein S. Making sense of possession states. Br J Hosp Med 1995; 53: 582.
10. Ward C. Possession and exorcism: psychopathology and psychotherapy in a magico-religious context. In: Ward C, ed. Altered states of consciousness and mental health. Thousand Oaks, CA: Sage Publications, 1989: 125–144.

SECTION VIII

Specific Conditions

ALCOHOL MISUSE

DEFINITION

The definition of drug or alcohol dependence includes at its core the desire or overwhelming urge or impulse to take the drug of choice, whether that is alcohol or a psychoactive drug. In addition to this strong desire, other features of dependence include difficulties in controlling substance-taking behaviour, withdrawal, tolerance, neglect of interests – and usually daily activities – and, lastly, persistence in taking the drug despite evidence of harm. These appear in both DSM-IV and ICD-10 criteria. However, the alcohol dependence syndrome as described by Edwards and Gross in 1976 contains slightly different features. In common with the other definitions, the alcohol dependence syndrome includes increased tolerance, repeated withdrawal and a subjective awareness of a compulsion to drink. Other criteria include a stereotyped pattern of drinking (the types of alcohol consumed become restricted and drinking becomes deeply ingrained), prominence or salience of drink-seeking behaviour (priority is given to acquiring and drinking alcohol), relief or avoidance of withdrawal by further drinking, and reinstatement of the syndrome after abstinence. The latter is often very striking, consumption of a single drink resulting in a rapid return to the person's previous level of drinking even after a significant period of abstinence.

While there are many similarities between dependence on alcohol and drugs in terms of their aetiology, prognosis and management, there are also some key differences. First, alcohol is a legal drug and is the most widely abused drug. Since those people dependent on illicit drugs will be acquiring them illegally, the percentage of people with antisocial or criminal personality traits is inevitably higher among illicit drug users than is seen in alcoholism.

Commonly misused illicit substances are cannabis, opiates, stimulants, hypnotics and tranquillizers, hallucinogens and solvents. Prescription medications such as opiates or benzodiazepines can also be abused. Although the specific physical and psychiatric complications may vary, the general principles underlying the management of dependency are the same for alcohol and drugs.

CLINICAL FEATURES OF ALCOHOL DEPENDENCY

Alcohol is a CNS depressant. While there is no specific alcohol receptor, alcohol affects many neurotransmitter systems, resulting in enhancement of inhibitory activity and reduction of excitatory activity in the brain.

PSYCHIATRIC COMPLICATIONS

These fall into several groups. Since alcohol is a legal and easily available drug, many people use alcohol to self-medicate their symptoms. The most common comorbid disorders are anxiety and depression, although patients may also suffer from psychosis or dementia. These pre-existing disorders need to be borne in mind once an alcohol-dependent person is abstinent, since failure to treat them adequately will inevitably result in a high relapse rate. The second group of disorders result from the abuse of alcohol; these include anxiety and depression but also importantly disorders such as Wernicke–Korsakoff encephalopathy and dementia. In addition, as a complication of withdrawal, delirium tremens may present with psychiatric symptoms.

ANXIETY DISORDERS

Alcohol abuse and dependence are associated with anxiety disorders in up to 30% of cases. The use of alcohol to overcome social anxiety and other phobias is a common route to heavy drinking and dependence. Notably, the incidence of anxiety, particularly panic disorder, may increase with continued drinking and dependence.

The majority of people dependent on alcohol experience symptoms of anxiety during the first few days of abstinence. These should resolve. Persistence of such symptoms or evidence of pre-existing anxiety disorder requires treatment using protocols as described above for anxiety disorders. Benzodiazepines should not, however, be used in this population – or, at least, only with extreme caution – because of the probable development of dependence.

DEPRESSION

As with anxiety, depressive symptoms are very common in alcohol abuse and dependence. Undoubtedly, alcohol significantly contributes to symptoms associated with depression. Again, similarly to anxiety, many of the symptoms resolve as the length of abstinence increases. Generally, if the depressive symptoms persist after 2–3 weeks of abstinence, treatment for depression should be started, following the usual protocols. While many clinicians feel that depression results from alcohol abuse, a recent review has shown that pre-existing depression is as likely as depression consequent upon alcohol dependence.

Suicide deserves particular mention, since about 25% of alcohol-dependent individuals attempt suicide. In addition, alcohol is often consumed in non-dependent people as part of their overdose. It is often a difficult clinical situation when a person presents intoxicated with alcohol (or drugs) and threatening suicide. The key to deciding how to manage this patient is exploring their past history to find out whether this is a change in their behaviour.

EATING DISORDERS

Although community surveys show that the rate of coexistence of eating disorders and alcohol dependence is not be very high – approximately 1%, in specialist centres – it does occur in up to 30% of people. Bulimia is more common than anorexia. In treating the patient, usually a young woman, attention should be paid to the relationship between the alcohol dependence and the eating disorder, since control of one often means reduced control of the other. These disorders have a similar psychological under-pinning but the initial goal should be abstinence from alcohol, given the lack of therapeutic efficacy of both pharmacotherapy and psychological strategies for managing eating disorders in the presence of alcohol abuse.

ALCOHOLIC HALLUCINOSIS

Alcoholic hallucinosis is characterized by third-person auditory hallucinations in clear consciousness. The content is usually derogatory or commanding. Usually, the onset of hallucinations is associated with withdrawal or at least reduction in the amount of alcohol consumed. More rarely, they arise in a person still drinking. Important in the differential diagnosis would be a psychotic illness or delirium tremens. While the condition usually resolves completely within 6 months, neuroleptics may be required to control symptoms. Some patients find them very distressing. Progression to a schizophrenic illness is associated with an increased family history of psychosis and occurs in about 5–20%.

PATHOLOGICAL JEALOUSY (OTHELLO SYNDROME)

This is characterized by development of a belief, usually delusional, although it may be overvalued, that the patient's partner or spouse has been unfaithful. This is twice as common in male alcoholics as in female alcoholics. Such a belief can result in a person searching for proof of the infidelity by following their partner, checking their clothes, diaries, etc. This, together with increased suspicion and interrogation of the partner, can often precipitate aggression and, in extreme cases, murder. Risk assessment is therefore crucial, particularly identifying any past history of violence. Separation from the partner may be required.

ALCOHOLIC DEMENTIA/COGNITIVE IMPAIRMENT

Some degree of cognitive impairment is very common in people with alcohol dependence or abuse presenting for treatment. Commonly, people describe problems with memory, which are often more problems of concentration than problems with recall. Abstinence results in significant improvement in the majority of people in all domains of cognition. Alcoholics may be less aware of impaired cognitive performance because of frontal lobe damage, the area of the brain most commonly affected. This manifests itself as impaired problem solving, planning, sequencing of behaviour, initiation, temporal order, judgement and aspects of personality including drive, motivation and inhibition. Obviously, these are all skills needed to initiate and maintain abstinence and the possibility of frontal lobe damage should therefore be considered if a patient is failing to adhere to treatment strategies. The mini-mental state can be used to screen for any areas of cognitive impairment. In addition, a full dementia screen, including MRI or CT scan, should be performed. Checking the patient's nutritional status is also of paramount importance, including prescribing thiamine.

AMNESIA

'Alcoholic blackouts' are periods of retrograde amnesia usually resulting from a period of intoxication.

KORSAKOFF'S SYNDROME AND WERNICKE'S ENCEPHALOPATHY

These are considered to be part of the same syndrome, in that Wernicke's is the more acute form with Korsakoff's developing later. There is increasing acknowledgement that Wernicke's encephalopathy is more common than was previously thought and may occur without the constellation of classical symptoms. Therefore, a high index of suspicion is required when assessing any alcoholic patient.

Deficiency of thiamine is implicated in the aetiology of both these disorders, which is why it is critical that this vitamin is given to any alcoholic. Unfortunately, alcoholics are generally poorly nourished, ingesting less thiamine; in addition, their stomachs are less able to absorb it. Therefore, if Wernicke's encephalopathy is suspected, parenteral replacement therapy should be instituted. Oral thiamine 100–200 mg per day is generally sufficient and should routinely be given with detoxification. Parenteral administration, however, has been associated with anaphylactic reactions and should therefore be performed in a hospital under supervision.

Clinical features of Wernicke's encephalopathy classically include confusion or clouded consciousness, nystagmus and ocular palsies, ataxia and peripheral neuropathy. Also associated may be gastrointestinal disturbances such as nausea and vomiting, some memory problems and emotional lability, with anxiety and insomnia. Post-mortem examinations have revealed acute degenerative changes in the diencephalon (hypothalamus, mammillary bodies), i.e. structures surrounding the third and fourth ventricles. In addition, parts of the cerebellum are affected. Examination of the tissue reveals petechial haemorrhages with astrocytic proliferation. Wernicke's encephalopathy has been reported to have a high morbidity of around 20%, with over 80% developing Korsakoff's syndrome.

Korsakoff's syndrome (or psychosis) shows neuropathology in similar areas to Wernicke's encephalopathy; however, reduced size of the mammillary bodies is no longer thought to be pathognomonic. Features of Korsakoff's syndrome classically include impairment of short-term memory, confabulation and sometime peripheral neuropathy. Confabulation is the falsification of memory in clear consciousness. Thus, when one speaks to a person with Korsakoff's syndrome they can present quite a convincing history but the events they describe are often impossible, e.g. serving in the Navy at a date when they would have been aged 6. The confabulation and impaired short-term memory occur with relative preservation of other intellectual functions and in clear consciousness, thus enabling the differentiation from both delirium and other forms of dementia. Korsakoff's syndrome is caused not only by alcoholism but by any causes of low thiamine, e.g. malnutrition, cancer of the stomach, persistent vomiting, carbon monoxide poisoning and a tumour in the region of the third ventricle. Since only approximately 20% of patients with Korsakoff's psychosis show any improvement when treated with thiamine, prevention of this disorder is critical.

PATHOLOGICAL DRUNKENNESS (*MANIE À POTU*)

This disorder said to occur in vulnerable individuals after drinking minute quantities of alcohol and is manifest as behavioural disturbance and disinhibition.

PROBLEMS ASSOCIATED WITH ALCOHOL WITHDRAWAL

Seizures

These commonly occur about 48 hours after alcohol has been consumed. Their incidence is increased in the presence of physical illness, hypoglycaemia, head injury, etc. The incidence of seizures rises as the number of detoxifications increases.

Delirium tremens

Delirium tremens is a severe form of alcohol withdrawal syndrome. It is a confusional state that arises generally between the second and fourth day after stopping drinking alcohol. This syndrome can present in people with enforced abstinence from alcohol such as those admitted to hospital who did not disclose their level of drinking. Patients often refer to having 'had the DTs' when they have merely suffered from severe but less problematic forms of withdrawal such as shakes or sweating, so taking a good history is important. The features of delirium tremens include clouding of consciousness, disorientation, tremor, autonomic overarousal, altered motor activity, mood instability (particularly anxiety, fear and paranoia) and insomnia. Hallucinations usually also occur and are classically small, mobile, coloured and often of animals. Auditory hallucinations may also be present and tend to be paranoid in nature. Delirium tremens is more likely in alcoholics suffering from physical illnesses such as metabolic disturbance or infection and dehydration. This disorder needs rapid treatment with benzodiazepines, which may have to be given intravenously, and treatment of any coexisting medical disorder. Delirium tremens occurs in 5–10% of patients, who are then at greater risk of repeated episodes. Mortality is about 10%. In addition to adequate sedation, parenteral vitamins should also be given.

Physical complications

Excessive consumption of alcohol results in increased morbidity and mortality because of the effects on a number of organ systems in the body. Increase in vulnerability is associated with increasing age, female sex, binge drinking and the total amount consumed. It is commonly forgotten that misuse of alcohol increases vulnerability to many cancers and cardiovascular disorders.

Gastrointestinal disorders

Commonly, most patients describe indigestion, reflecting oesophagitis, gastritis and ulceration. A Mallory–Weiss tear may be seen after a heavy bout of drinking.

The liver

Alcohol is the commonest cause of liver damage in the UK. The first change resulting from alcohol abuse is deposits of fat in the liver, leading to fatty liver. This is generally asymptomatic, although the patient may present with an enlarged tender liver. It is present in up to 90% of heavy drinkers. Liver function tests (gamma GT, AST, ALT, ALP) will be abnormal. Fatty liver is reversible with abstinence. The next stage of liver disease is alcoholic hepatitis, which can range from being asymptomatic through to aggressive hepatitis and death. Without abstinence, hepatitis usually progresses to cirrhosis. This severe end of the spectrum is manifest as loss of appetite, abdominal pain, nausea and vomiting, and jaundice. Between 8% and 30% of heavy drinkers develop cirrhosis. There are differences in vulnerability, with a possible genetic influence, and females are more vulnerable. Cirrhosis is associated with the deposit of fibrous tissue in the liver resulting in liver dysfunction (abnormal liver function test, including clotting). In addition, as a consequence of the scarring, blood flow through the liver is reduced, resulting in increased pressure in the portal vessels. This so-called portal hypertension can, in turn, cause bleeding from veins at the lower end of the oesophagus (oesophageal varices), which can be fatal. Patients with limited cirrhosis, once they stop drinking, will have no further progression of the disease. Patients with liver failure may be considered for a liver transplant. All these alcoholic liver diseases are further complicated by coexisting hepatitis B and/or C. Screening should therefore always be performed.

Cardiovascular disorders

Alcohol intoxication may result in an arrhythmia. Alcohol may also induce heart muscle disease (alcoholic cardiomyopathy). Population-based epidemiological studies have shown that drinking small amounts of alcohol appears to be protective against coronary heart disease. However, drinking above the recommended level is associated with an increased risk of hypertension, atherosclerosis and stroke.

Metabolic disorders

Hypoglycaemia can be seen with alcohol intoxication; alcoholic ketoacidosis is more rarely seen and usually arises after an alcoholic binge. Gout may occur.

Musculoskeletal

Chronic alcoholic myopathy is quite common and predominantly affects proximal muscles, particularly in the legs. Osteoporosis may be seen. Dupuytren's contracture is also associated with alcoholism.

Haematological disorders

Macrocytosis (increased MCV) is common. Folate and vitamin B_{12} deficiency may contribute. Anaemia, neutropenia and thrombocytopenia may also occur.

Respiratory disorders

Heavy drinking and alcohol dependency are associated with an increased incidence of pulmonary infections. Tuberculosis is on the increase in the UK and contributory factors include the poor conditions many alcoholics live in, poor nutrition and also the fact that alcohol suppresses the immune system. Importantly, many drinkers are also heavy smokers.

Neurological complications

- **Marchiafava–Bignami syndrome**: this condition is characterized by ataxia, epilepsy, dysarthria and impaired consciousness. The underlying neuropathology includes demyelination of the corpus callosum
- **Central pontine myelinosis**: patients generally present with nausea and vomiting, leading to confusion and coma. Associated symptoms are pseudobulbar palsy, quadriplegia and loss of sensation in the limbs and trunk. The condition is often fatal
- **Alcoholic cerebellar degeneration**: this disorder generally presents with ataxic gait and incoordination of the legs. The cerebellum appears quite sensitive to the effects of alcohol. In addition to the direct toxic effect of alcohol, nutritional difficulties may also be an important factor

Fetal alcohol syndrome

It is clear that alcohol can cause fetal damage; however, the quantity of alcohol that results in such damage is still debated. There are gradations within fetal alcohol syndrome but they all include a small head with shortened eyelids, underdeveloped upper lip, maxillary hypoplasia and flattened wide nose, short stature, cognitive impairment and underdeveloped mental delay.

Social sequelae

Patients who have a problem with alcohol commonly present with many social problems, some as a consequence of financial difficulties. Areas that should be probed include family, work, housing, financial difficulties and forensic issues, including drink driving. Drink driving has a high profile in the UK. Patients should be specifically asked whether they drive when they know they are over the limit and, if misuse of alcohol is suspected, they should be advised to inform the Driver and Vehicle Licensing Authority (DVLA). In some situations, e.g. if they persist in driving over the limit or their job involves driving, you can inform the DVLA if they have ignored your advice. The many social sequelae of alcoholism or misuse of alcohol can usually be best tackled once abstinence has been achieved. A multidisciplinary approach with involvement of social services and local advisory organizations is appropriate.

TREATMENT OF ALCOHOL DEPENDENCE

Managing withdrawal

It is likely, if somebody is dependent on alcohol, that they will require pharmacological cover of their withdrawal from it. Generally, if in doubt, medication should be offered. The next decision is whether detoxification can be achieved in the community or whether it requires inpatient admission. Reasons for inpatient admission include previous severe withdrawal symptoms such as seizures and delirium tremens, lack of home support, physical debility, coexisting psychiatric illness and a history of previous failed community detoxification. Generally, dedicated inpatient beds for detoxification are not widely available, so patients can be admitted to either a general psychiatric ward or a medical bed if one is available. Most patients can be safely detoxified at home but they should be warned what to expect and a plan for their first few days to weeks of abstinence should be in place prior to detoxification.

In an outpatient setting a reducing dose of a benzodiazepine, generally chlordiazepoxide (e.g. 20 mg four times daily) should be prescribed. Daily prescribing in conjunction with breathalizing the patient is a common strategy. This reduces the likelihood of patients taking their reducing regime either inappropriately or with alcohol. Clomethiazole should not be used because of its greater addictive potential and risk of fatal respiratory depression if taken with alcohol. In addition, thiamine 100–200 mg daily should be prescribed. Inpatient detoxification can follow a similar protocol but it is easier to titrate the chlordiazepoxide dose to cover symptoms adequately.

The aim of pharmacological cover for alcohol withdrawal is to prevent severe complications such as fits and delirium tremens. The use of anticonvulsants to prevent fits is routine in some clinics, although the evidence suggesting that it does reduce seizure incidence is unclear.

Maintaining abstinence

There are many different strategies employed in helping people to remain abstinent from alcohol. Fortunately, this can mean that, if a person has failed with one strategy, an alternative one can be used. As with any therapy, a key aspect is the relationship between therapist and patient.

Therapies can either be individual or administered on a group basis. It is critical that any comorbid disorders should also be adequately treated. The best known organization that helps alcoholics is Alcoholics Anonymous (AA). Enshrined in AA are 'the 12 steps' through which alcoholics must move in their recovery. These principles have been incorporated in the Minnesota model, which is prevalent in many rehabilitation settings. Many alcoholics say they do not like AA because of its religious overtones. While this may be true of some groups, it is not always the case and the patient's motivation should be further explored. Relapse prevention, cognitive behavioural strategies and motivational interviewing are currently widely used in treatment settings.

Increasingly, pharmacotherapy is employed to help maintain abstinence. Currently, acamprosate is licensed in the UK and naltrexone can also be used.

Acamprosate probably inhibits *N*-methyl D-aspartate (NMDA) function, although its exact mechanism is unclear. It has been shown to double the rate of abstinence to about 20% at 6 months. Unfortunately it is not clear who will respond to acamprosate, although those with anxiety symptoms may be more likely to benefit.

Naltrexone is an opiate antagonist and appears to block the positive reinforcing effects of alcohol. It is more widely used in the US, where similar results to acamprosate have been obtained. If a person drinks alcohol while taking either of these two drugs there is evidence that they will drink less and stop sooner.

Often, alcoholics are perceived as a difficult group of patients to treat; however, their attendance rate and ability to comply with treatment are not very different from those of patients with other relapsing remitting disorders. Unfortunately, relapse is part of the condition and a plan to be implemented in the event of relapse should also be part of treatment.

ILLICIT DRUG USE

There are often regional differences in what kinds of drug are abused. The effect of any drug depends not only on the drug itself but also on characteristics of the person (e.g. mood, personality) and the environmental setting in which the drug was taken. In addition, the route of administration is important, since the faster the drug gets into the brain the more reinforcing or addictive it will be. Thus smoking crack is more addictive than injecting cocaine, which is more addictive than chewing coca leaves. The short duration of the effect of crack cocaine compared to intravenous cocaine means that repeated administration is necessary to maintain any effect.

It is hard to get an exact figure of how many people are using illicit drugs. Although the Home Office Addicts Index is no longer active, regional drug misuse databases are maintained. The 1996 OPCS survey showed a prevalence rate of 2.2% for drug dependence. There was increasing use of illicit drugs in young school-age children.

OPIATE MISUSE

Clinical features of opiate dependency

There are a large number of opiate derivatives that may be abused, including morphine, heroin (diamorphine), pethidine, dihydrocodeine, buprenorphine and methadone. It must be remembered, when calculating any substitution prescription, that the purity of street heroin varies widely. The prevalence of heroin use is thought to be less than 1% within the UK; however its abuse has a high profile because of the criminality associated with it.

Opiates produce a variety of physical and psychological changes, including mood change, euphoria and intense pleasure, drowsiness and sleep, analgesia, reduction in body temperature, pupillary restriction, respiratory and cough reflex suppression, reduced pulse rate and blood pressure, and nausea and vomiting. In particular, pupillary size is a good clinical sign of opiate use. Heroin may initially be smoked ('chasing the dragon'), then injected subcutaneously ('skin popping'), followed by intravenous use.

An opiate addict is commonly abusing or dependent on other drugs, such as benzodiazepines, alcohol or stimulants such as cocaine. A comprehensive drug history is required to elicit the role drugs play in the addict's life to set out an appropriate treatment strategy.

Comorbidity or dual diagnosis

As with alcohol abuse, many patients with drug dependence have a comorbid psychiatric disorder. Many patients have used drugs as medication for their psychiatric problems, or at least drug use appears to be associated with the emergence of such problems. It is often difficult to tease out cause or consequence. Identification of any comorbid diagnosis is important, since these patients have a poorer prognosis, more hospitalizations, poorer compliance with treatment, relative neuroleptic unresponsiveness and increased rates of forensic problems and homelessness. In many parts of the country there are local strategies to develop services for those with dual diagnosis. The comorbid disorder should be treated by the usual protocols, although the interplay with drug use is also obviously of paramount importance and must be also addressed.

Criminality

Since many drug addicts come to the attention of services via the legal system, there are now many treatment options available either in prison or as an alternative to a custodial sentence. Early signs suggest that these strategies reduce the risk of returning to use and to criminal activity. It must be remembered that drugs such as heroin are widely available in most prisons, with increased risks such as greater needle sharing.

Mortality

Drug addicts have an increased mortality rate. Death from overdose of opiates is not uncommon; many addicts report that they know someone who has died in these circumstances. Deaths often occur after a period of abstinence, when the addict's tolerance is much reduced. In addition, death may occur if the purity of street heroin is much higher than the addict is used to. Lastly, the combination of opiates with other drugs such as alcohol or benzodiazepines makes respiratory depression more likely. If an opiate overdose is suspected, naloxone, an opiate antagonist, should be given either intravenously or intramuscularly. The half-life of naloxone is shorter than that of heroin or other opiates and the patient will therefore need to be monitored. Naloxone may have to be administered again.

Physical complications

Many physical effects of opiates are predictable from the known effects described above. Patients are often also physically debilitated because of poor nutrition or homelessness, so infections are more common. These include bacterial endocarditis, septicaemia, tuberculosis, pneumonia and brain abscesses. Problems of aspiration of vomit may occur through vomiting while respiratorily distressed. Cardiac arrhythmias are also seen. Myopathy may occur; rhabdomyolysis causes renal damage. Many infections are secondary to the patient's injecting behaviour; hence skin abscesses are commonly seen and injection sites should be checked (wherever in the body they may be). In addition to the infections above, the patient may suffer from osteomyelitis and transverse myelitis.

If the person has been injecting, it is likely that they have shared needles or equipment, e.g. spoons or syringes. The risk of transmission of hepatitis B and C and human immunodeficiency virus (HIV) is therefore high. Vaccination against hepatitis B can be offered if available. A significant proportion of opiate addicts also abuse alcohol or are alcohol-dependent. This will need to be addressed as well, particularly if they are hepatitis-B- and/or hepatitis-C-positive.

The spread of HIV provided an impetus for treatment programmes to aim at 'harm minimization' rather than purely abstinence. Thus, needle exchanges where addicts could obtain clean needles became more common and stabilization on substitute drugs such as methadone was advocated. Such strategies prevented or at least reduced the risk of infection with HIV or hepatitis B/C, since the addict's use of heroin was either dramatically reduced or at least involved clean needles.

Social sequelae

These can be very similar to problems associated with alcohol dependency. However, there is a particular association between illicit drug use and crime, primarily because of the necessity of obtaining large sums of money to maintain a habit. The most common crimes are types of theft such as burglary and shoplifting. Women in particular, but also men, may act as prostitutes. Some addicts maintain their habit by supplying drugs. Engagement in treatment services and stabilization on drugs such as methadone is associated with a reduction in crime. Such a decrease in associated criminality has also been a key aim of harm minimization strategies.

TREATMENT

Stabilization and harm minimization

This pragmatic approach is used to prevent secondary sequelae from drug use such as infections and crime. Engaging somebody in treatment with substitute prescribing also allows time for a better therapeutic relationship to be built, time for education on risks of drug abuse and secondary activities such as safer sex, and time to treat any physical or psychiatric problems. Lastly, motivational interviewing can be used to prepare the addict to change their addictive behaviour and move towards abstinence.

Methadone is the most commonly prescribed substitute therapy. It is generally taken once a day, although addicts might want to take it twice a day. Obviously, methadone has a street value and ways of trying to avoid 'street diversion' include supervised consumption, either at the treatment centre or at the pharmacy. Patients usually 'graduate' to 'take-home' supplies or prescription of enough for days to weeks once they engage in services. In addition, young children have died from consuming methadone, so parents should be appropriately counselled.

Generally, on first contact with services, an addict is stabilized on a substitute such as methadone so that their use of street opiates is stopped or at least minimized. An addict should have a positive urine for opiates before they are started on methadone. It is usually safe to begin with up to 50 mg of methadone. As a rough guide, 40 mg of methadone (1 mg/ml mixture) is approximately equivalent to 0.5 g of street heroin. Most addicts stabilize on a dose of methadone between 60 mg and 80 mg, although some receive far less and others far more.

Newer substitute therapies are now available, including buprenorphine and LAAM. Buprenorphine has a critical advantage over methadone in that it is safe in overdose, and heroin, if taken on top, will have no pharmacological effects because the opiate receptors are blocked by buprenorphine, which is a partial opiate agonist. LAAM has a longer half-life than methadone and therefore only needs to be taken once every 2–3 days. This is important if the substitute is given under 'supervised consumption', since the patient needs to attend the service less often.

Managing opiate withdrawal

Unlike alcohol withdrawal, opiate withdrawal is not life-threatening. The syndrome generally appears within hours after the last heroin dose, peaking at 2–3 days. Often, the addict is acutely sensitive to withdrawal symptoms, which drive further opiate use. Characteristic symptoms of withdrawal include agitation, lacrimation, rhinorrhoea, abdominal cramps and diarrhoea, sweating with goose bumps, aching muscles and joints, yawning and insomnia.

If a patient is dependent on opiates and asks for detoxification, assessment is required as to whether this is the correct objective. It may be that maintenance might be a more appropriate option, with the aim of harm minimization (see above). Attempting detoxification while using opiates on top of their methadone prescription suggests that the patient is not ready for abstinence. As with alcohol dependency, the first consideration is whether detoxification can be achieved as an inpatient or an outpatient. Many detoxifications are carried out on an outpatient basis but, as with alcohol dependency, failure to manage community detoxification, physical illness, pregnancy, HIV infection or high-risk living situations would suggest that inpatient detoxification is required. Withdrawal during pregnancy is best undertaken in the second trimester.

There are several ways of weaning someone from opiates. Whether methadone or buprenorphine is being used as a substitute, detoxification may involve gradual reduction of the dose of substitute opiate. This may take weeks to months. Reducing the dose of opiates is not the only way of ameliorating signs of withdrawal. Many symptoms, such as sweating, rhinorrhoea, agitation, insomnia and increased arousal, are secondary to increased noradrenergic activity. These can be ameliorated by lofexidine, an α_2-agonist that does not cause significant hypertension, unlike its predecessor, clonidine. Varying protocols are used but a rapidly increased dose of lofexidine can be 'dovetailed' with a rapidly (e.g. over 2 days) reduced dose of methadone. Other drugs that ameliorate gastrointestinal symptoms and insomnia may routinely be offered. Lofexidine is increasingly used in the community.

Maintenance of abstinence

As with alcohol dependence, detoxification is only the first step. There are many different approaches, including relapse prevention, motivational interviewing and cognitive behavioural strategies, whether in a one-to-one setting, involving partners or families, or in groups. Programmes using the 12-step or Minnesota model are available. With the declining availability of inpatient units in the UK, the majority of residential provision is in the voluntary or non-statutory sector. Depending on the region, these are arranged through social services and may depend on self-referral by the addict.

Naltrexone, an opiate antagonist, is also available to help people remain abstinent. This works by blocking any effects of taking opiates. Prior to starting, a naloxone challenge should be performed to check that the patient is opiate-free. In programmes based on the 12-step model, use of naltrexone is somewhat controversial, since taking another drug to remain 'clean' can be interpreted as using a 'prop' instead of working on one's problems oneself.

Prognosis and outcome

Opiate addiction is associated with a mortality of 1–2%, suicide and accidental overdose accounting for up to half of all deaths in opiate addicts. Whichever treatment strategy is used, it is clear that the longer the patient stays in contact with services the better the outcome. Poorer prognosis is associated with psychiatric comorbidity, including personality disorder, other dependencies, including alcohol, and forensic involvement. For many addicts, abstinence is not a realistic option, especially if drug use persists into their thirties.

STIMULANT MISUSE

Amphetamines

Clinical features

Amphetamines are also known as 'speed' or 'whizz' and stimulate the release of dopamine and inhibit its reuptake. They can be taken in tablet form, snorted or injected. In some parts of the UK, amphetamines are widely abused. They may be used (e.g. by students studying for exams) in order to stay awake longer, or as an aid to weight reduction. Like all stimulants, amphetamines tend to be used in binges with many drug-free days. The effects of amfetamine and other stimulants include euphoria, energy and heightened alertness. In addition, they tend to make people more verbal and not to appear to need food or sleep. Their use, however, is also associated with agitation and irritability leading to psychotic symptoms such as paranoia and hallucinations. Stimulant intoxication is therefore included in the differential diagnosis for a person presenting as psychotic. If the psychosis is drug-induced, physiological signs such as raised blood pressure and pulse, dilated pupils, sweating and tremor may be present.

Treatment

Withdrawal from amphetamines and stimulants after chronic use is associated with dysphoria, anhedonia, fatigue, reduced energy, hyperphagia and sleep disturbance caused by hypersomnia. Depression can be the most troubling problem and it has been suggested that withdrawal should be covered with an antidepressant. Some centres may offer substitute amfetamine prescribing, although this is controversial and is only conducted in specialist centres.

Cocaine

Clinical features

Cocaine is a potent blocker of dopamine reuptake sites. The most common route of administration is snorting. Cocaine can also be injected, either alone or with heroin ('speed ball'). Cocaine, whether injected or snorted, has to circulate within the body before reaching the brain. The freed alkaloid base or 'crack' can be smoked and hence reaches the brain faster. This faster rate of onset, and therefore offset, results in a higher addictive potential because of the rapidity of the on/off effect. Its effects are similar to those of amfetamine.

Like amfetamine, cocaine has been used to increase confidence and improve work performance. Because of its very short half-life, cocaine or crack is often taken many times in a session and can cost many hundreds or thousands of pounds. Similarly to amfetamine, intoxication is associated with autonomic arousal, agitation and psychosis.

Treatment

There are few treatment centres dealing solely with stimulant abuse and, as with amphetamines, there is relatively little role for pharmacotherapy. At one time, desipramine was advocated to prevent the 'cocaine crash' – the depression that ensues after stopping taking cocaine. It is not clear that antidepressants are of any help. Currently, there are many strategies and developments, including cocaine vaccines, but it is likely that psychological strategies such as motivational interviewing and cognitive therapy will remain the mainstay of treatment.

Ecstasy

Clinical features

Ecstasy (3,4-methylene dioxymethamfetamine, MDMA) is a stimulant with greater hallucinogenic properties than either amfetamine or cocaine. Its primary mode of action is to inhibit the reuptake of monoamines, particularly 5-HT (serotonin). There is evidence from animal studies to show that Ecstasy is selectively neurotoxic to serotonergic neurones but whether the same is true in man remains controversial. Acutely, Ecstasy causes an increase in empathy, sensuality and energy. Less positive effects include anxiety and psychosis, particularly paranoia. Many psychiatric symptoms have been described following Ecstasy use and in some cases these are due to other illicit substances included in the tablets – amfetamine, ketamine, etc.

Generally, Ecstasy is taken at weekends in clubs. There is now a clear associated feeling of depression 2–3 days after, i.e. 'midweek blues'. In addition, there have been documented facts on cognitive performance and memory. The number of Ecstasy-related deaths has a high profile in the UK. Causes have included inappropriate antidiuretic hormone (ADH) secretion, which, in combination with excessive drinking to combat the hyperthermia induced by the drug, has resulted in cerebral oedema.

Treatment

This is as for other stimulants.

Phencyclidine and ketamine (angel dust)

Both drugs were developed as anaesthetics, and ketamine is still used as one. Both drugs cause analgesia and amnesia and, at higher doses, can cause excitement, hallucinations, delusions, paranoia, disorientation and lack of judgement. Both ketamine and phencyclidine are NMDA antagonists. Overdose of either drug can cause seizures and coma.

Hallucinogens – LSD and mescaline

Lysergic acid ethlamide (LSD) was extremely popular in the 1960s but then fell out of common use. However its use is on the increase again. LSD affects the serotonergic system, primarily acting as an agonist of 5-HT_2 receptors. It is generally taken orally as 'tabs' – squares of blotting paper on which LSD has been absorbed. The most common experiences are marked perceptual distortion with visual illusions and hallucinations. There is usually an altered state of awareness, with euphoria, which can result in inappropriate behaviour that may put the person at risk. Visual hallucinations are more common than other modalities and people describe synaesthesia, i.e. colours are heard, sounds are seen.

Adverse effects of LSD include sympathetic overdrive. The best known adverse event, which happens in about 15% of people, is 'flashbacks' – a recurrence of part of an original LSD experience. Notably, it may occur up to some years after the original use of the drug and is usually the recurrence of a 'bad trip'.

It may therefore manifest as a highly anxious state. Such an episode may respond to simple support, but medication such as sedatives may be required.

Benzodiazepines

Clinical features

Benzodiazepines enhance GABAergic function and hence increase inhibitory activity in the brain. They are sedative, hypnotic, anxiolytic, anticonvulsant and amnesic. Dependence can result from illicit use only or from prescribed drugs. Tolerance can develop after several weeks and hence prolonged prescription (> 2 weeks) is not recommended. Risk factors for the development of tolerance and dependence include a history of drug dependence, high doses of benzodiazepines with a short half-life, and psychiatric problems such as dysphoria and insomnia. Prevention of dependence by avoiding prescription in vulnerable people is vital.

Treatment

Benzodiazepine withdrawal frequently includes anxiety, insomnia, restlessness, agitation, irritability and muscle tension. These generally occur within days of stopping benzodiazepines and resolve by 2 weeks. Such withdrawal symptoms may be a re-emergence of the underlying psychopathology if benzodiazepines were prescribed to begin with. Less frequent presentations are nausea, sweating, lethargy, hyperacusis, nightmares, ataxia, blurred vision and, rarely, psychosis, seizures, tinnitus and paranoid delusions.

In order to avoid these problems, conversion from a short half-life benzodiazepine to diazepam, which has a long half-life, is the first step. Conversion tables are available. Diazepam can then be tapered off over many weeks to months, if necessary.

Cannabis

Clinical features

This drug is the most commonly abused illicit drug. The primary active constituent is δ-9 tetrahydrocannibol (THC) but different sources of cannabis can have other active forms. There are cannabis receptors widely distributed in the brain. Cannabis is generally smoked, either in a pure form or with tobacco, or consumed by eating or drinking as a tea. Its use results in mild euphoria, relaxation, enhanced perceptual awareness and distorted time awareness. Other effects include impaired concentration, attention, short-term memory and motor function. Unpleasant effects such as anxiety, paranoia and dysphoria can occur. There is evidence that highly potent cannabis can result in psychosis, which generally abates on abstinence and occurs in those with a family history of psychosis. A causal link to schizophrenia is still debated. Cannabis dependence is now recognized. Whether chronic cannabis use results in 'brain damage' still remains unclear. Heavy smoking, however, probably does result in an increase in pulmonary damage, including cancer, since a cannabis joint contains more tar and is inhaled more deeply than a 'normal' cigarette.

SCHIZOPHRENIA

DEFINITION

The most common psychotic disorder, schizophrenia is characterized by abnormalities in perception, beliefs, thought processing and expression, volition and reality testing. The phenomenology of schizophrenia can be divided into acute and chronic features.

CLINICAL FEATURES

Acute illness

- **AUDITORY HALLUCINATIONS**
  Although both second- and third-person auditory hallucinations occur, it is the latter that are of diagnostic importance. Third-person auditory hallucinations are characteristically described as two or more people discussing the patient, often in a derogatory manner; also experienced is third-person commentary, in which patients hear someone describing their actions as they are carried out, and *echo de la pensée*, in which patients hear their own thoughts aloud
- **SOMATIC (BODILY) HALLUCINATIONS**
  Although diagnostically significant, these are less common than auditory hallucinations
- **DELUSIONAL BELIEFS**
  These are very common, particularly those with persecutory content. The most important diagnostically, and also the rarest, are primary delusions, in which a fully formed belief suddenly occurs 'out of the blue'. Ideas of reference are also very common in schizophrenia; unrelated notices, signs or remarks are believed to be messages with specific meaning for the patient. Ideas of reference are often found in the media, and usually have a tangential connection with the subject
- **THOUGHT INSERTION/WITHDRAWAL/BROADCAST**
  Here the patient believes that others know what they are thinking, either because their thoughts can be heard aloud (akin to *echo de la pensée*) or because they are transmitted through radio or television. This feature probably represents both delusional beliefs and auditory hallucinations
- **PASSIVITY EXPERIENCES**
  In these the patient feels that their bodily functions, emotions or thoughts are under external control. The most important experience diagnostically is thought block, in which a train of thought comes to a sudden halt, accompanied by the experience of having the thought removed from the patient's mind
- **FORMAL THOUGHT DISORDER**
  Here, the individual has difficulty expressing their own thoughts. In mild

thought disorder they have trouble maintaining a train of thought (loosening of association) and may appear to 'go off at a tangent' or talk past the point (*vorbeireden*). When more severe, this results in disjunctures in thought – 'knight's move' thinking (or derailment). When it is very severe, words become jumbled up in a 'word salad' (verbigeration), which may contain examples of words invented by the individual (neologisms)

- **MOOD**
  Individuals with acute schizophrenia may be highly suspicious, aroused and irritable, or grandiose

Chronic symptoms

Also referred to as 'negative symptoms', the symptoms of chronic schizophrenia include affective blunting, apathy, poverty of thought and speech, social withdrawal and self-neglect. Although the acute symptoms are extremely distressing, and may lead to potentially life-threatening behaviour, it is the chronic symptoms that are responsible for impairment and handicap.

EPIDEMIOLOGY

The lifetime risk of developing schizophrenia is about 1% in the general population. In the UK, the prevalence is about 0.5–1% and the incidence about 14:100 000 per year. There is no sex difference in prevalence. The first onset typically occurs between 15 and 45 years of age, although men exhibit symptoms earlier than women.

Prevalence is highest in low socioeconomic groups, among the unmarried and in urban areas. Although these findings have traditionally been explained in terms of 'social drift', this has been challenged by recent findings.

In the UK, rates in first-generation immigrants from the Caribbean are higher than in the indigenous population (about 2:1) but they are higher still in second-generation Afro-Caribbeans (about 10:1). The latter finding has yet to be explained.

Findings that support a neurodevelopmental model of schizophrenia are associations between schizophrenia and season of birth, obstetric complications and maternal exposure to either an influenza epidemic or starvation during the first and/or second trimester of pregnancy.

Despite similar rates of incidence around the world, the outcome of schizophrenia appears to be significantly better in developing countries than in North America or Europe.

BASIC SCIENCE

Recent developments in neuroimaging have established that there are structural and functional brain abnormalities in schizophrenia, although none are considered to be pathognomonic. Chief among the structural changes are lateral ventricular enlargement and a diminution in the size of the frontal lobes, particularly the amygdala, hippocampus and parahippocampal gyrus. Thickening of the corpus callosum has also been reported.

Important functional changes, detected by studies of local blood flow and neuronal activity, have demonstrated not only that there is reduced activity in the frontal lobes ('hypofrontality') but also that auditory hallucinations are associated with increased activity in Broca's area, a part of the brain normally associated with speech production. The advent of MRI, and more recently functional MRI, has led to a renewed interest in the neuroanatomy and neurophysiology of schizophrenia.

The dominant neuropharmacological model of schizophrenia is still based on the dopamine hypothesis, in which the symptoms of this disorder are accounted for by a relative excess of dopamine.

Twin and family studies indicate that there is a strong genetic component in the aetiology of schizophrenia. Concordance rates in monozygotic twins are about 50%, compared with 10% in dizygotic twins. The lifetime risk of schizophrenia is increased about 10-fold in siblings of probands, 12-fold in children of one schizophrenic parent and 50-fold in children of two schizophrenic parents. Adoption studies have found that the children of schizophrenics have significantly higher rates of schizophrenia than members of the family into which they are adopted. Results from molecular genetic studies indicate that the predisposition to schizophrenia is likely to involve several genes rather than just one.

It has been suggested that there are two aetiological 'types' of schizophrenia, one that is inherited ('genetic') and one that occurs because of a 'brain injury' suffered at a developmentally sensitive stage. Despite sound evidence of premorbid developmental abnormalities during childhood and adolescence, the 'neurodevelopmental' model of schizophrenia has yet to be substantiated.

DIFFERENTIAL DIAGNOSIS

ORGANIC

There is much debate about the relationship with drug-induced psychoses (especially LSD, Ecstasy, amphetamines and cocaine/crack). The differential diagnosis includes very rare conditions such as Huntington's chorea, Wilson's disease, temporal lobe epilepsy, frontal or temporal lobe tumour, early multiple sclerosis, early systemic lupus erythematosus and porphyria

PSYCHIATRIC

- **Mania**: although the symptoms often overlap, mania is characterized by a prominent affective component (elation, grandiosity, disinhibition, overactivity, irritability and lability of mood) while acute schizophrenia is characterized most often by suspicion, paranoia or perplexity
- **Schizoaffective disorder**: in ICD-10 this diagnosis requires that the person meets the criteria for both schizophrenia and a bipolar disorder
- **Depression**: chronic schizophrenia may mimic or coexist with depression, particularly in young people and those who retain insight into the nature of their illness

MANAGEMENT

Studies in the UK, Australia and the USA have shown that patients with both acute and chronic schizophrenia can be cared for satisfactorily outside traditional psychiatric hospital inpatient settings. However, while this community-based care has proved significantly less costly than inpatient treatment, and is preferred by patients and their carers, there is no evidence of any clinical or social outcome differences.

Management of acute schizophrenia

- The first priority is to ensure the safety of the patient and others. Schizophrenic patients are more likely to be the victims of violent crime than its perpetrators. Although rarely homicidal, patients with schizophrenia are at high risk of suicide, and careful assessment of risk is mandatory. This should involve discussion with informants
- The mainstay of treatment is pharmacological, in the form of neuroleptic drugs. These may be administered orally, intramuscularly or, in an emergency (to achieve rapid tranquillization), intravenously. The most sedating neuroleptic is chlorpromazine. Some patients may benefit from augmentation of neuroleptics with diazepam (for a short time) if aroused, lithium carbonate if associated with prominent affective symptoms, or carbamazepine if aggressive
- While most acute (positive) symptoms can be controlled with regular doses of the older neuroleptic drugs, some are resistant to such treatment, even at high doses. A proportion of these individuals will respond to newer antipsychotics, including risperidone and clozapine. The latter may sometimes produce dramatic results but requires careful monitoring because of the risk of agranulocytosis
- Psychoeducational and adherence-enhancing strategies are very important at this stage

Management of chronic schizophrenia

- Rehabilitation aims to allow the patient to lead as nearly normal a life as possible, and incorporates relapse prevention. Effective rehabilitation addresses all aspects of social, psychological and emotional functioning
- Relapse prevention may be achieved by (1) ensuring compliance with medication, (2) assertive aftercare coordinated by a keyworker and (3) support and education for relatives and other carers
- Since patients with schizophrenia often lack insight into their condition, many cease compliance with medication at the earliest opportunity. The use of depot injections is a partial solution, since it allows medication to be given only every 3–4 weeks. A recent development is the use of so-called motivational interviews to enhance insight and therefore compliance with medication

- Domiciliary visiting of patients who default from treatment or who fail to attend clinic appointments may increase the chance of compliance with medication but certainly facilitates early intervention when signs of relapse do occur
- There is very strong evidence that supportive psychoeducational family therapy can significantly reduce the rate of relapse, particularly in patients who are also compliant with prophylactic medication. The main aim of this type of treatment is to help families to understand more about this illness, and to minimize the chance of over-stimulation at home. Research indicates that criticism, over-involvement and prolonged face-to-face contact with other family members are all associated with high rates of both arousal and subsequent recurrence of psychotic symptoms
- Cognitive therapy has been shown to be of clear benefit
- Rehabilitation requires a formal assessment of: individual skills in activities of daily living (cooking, cleaning, washing, personal hygiene and budgeting), usually by an occupational therapist; housing and financial circumstances; and the availability, ability and attitudes of informal carers. Patients may need help with some or all of these; if severely disabled they may need to live in supported accommodation
- Previous models of rehabilitation incorporated graded hierarchies of residential and occupational settings through which individual patients would move when they were able. Day centres offering mixtures of structured occupational therapy and informal opportunities to socialize have largely replaced sheltered workshops. Most areas have a range of different types of supported accommodation, although most are owned and operated by voluntary organizations, such as housing associations, and are funded by social services and housing benefit payments. Supported accommodation ranges from nursing homes staffed 24 hours a day by qualified nurses, through hostels staffed by care assistants in which there may be a member of staff on site at night, to supported group homes or flats in which residents are visited by non-resident staff

AFFECTIVE DISORDERS

DEFINITION

Two types of mood disorder are recognized by categorical systems of classification – mania and depression – although in reality these probably exist as extremes on a continuum. Both ICD-10 and DSM-IV abound with different ways of classifying depression. For the present purposes we distinguish only between the psychotic disorders (manic-depressive psychosis and psychotic depression) and unipolar, non-psychotic depression. Although manic-depressive psychosis may first present with a manic episode, one or more episodes of depression invariably follow. 'Unipolar' mania is extremely uncommon.

CLINICAL FEATURES OF MANIA (ICD-10 F30)

Although described as a persistent excessive elevation of mood, patients suffering from mania commonly present in a so-called mixed affective state, with lability of mood and features of both 'classical' mania and depression. Manic episodes generally develop over 1–2 days, culminating in disinhibition, overactivity and increasingly uncontrollable behaviour. Patients with acute mania may do themselves great harm through overspending and sexual disinhibition, and are prone to physical exhaustion. Mania is by definition a psychotic condition.

- **ELEVATION OF MOOD**
  Characterized by overactivity, euphoria, grandiosity and increased libido
- **THOUGHT DISORDER**
  Including pressure of speech, flight of ideas, puns and clang associations (rhyming)
- **RESTLESSNESS, INSOMNIA AND IRRITABILITY, INTOLERANCE OF FRUSTRATION AND PERSISTENT DEMANDS**
  May lead to aggression and/or violence
- **LACK OF INSIGHT AND DIMINISHED JUDGEMENT**
  This, combined with the above symptoms, may lead to, for example, overspending or unprotected sexual intercourse, occurrences that may have consequences extending beyond the duration of the acute manic episode
- **HALLUCINATIONS**
  Most commonly auditory but also in other sensory modalities
- **DELUSIONAL BELIEFS AND IDEAS OF REFERENCE**
  Particularly involving grandiose and/or persecutory themes

Note that Schneider's first-rank symptoms of schizophrenia occur in about 20% of patients with mania.

CLINICAL FEATURES OF DEPRESSION (ICD-10 F32)

In contrast to mania, depression is only rarely associated with psychotic symptoms. The signs and symptoms of depression are often considered under the following headings.

- **PHYSICAL (OR 'VEGETATIVE')**
  - **Poor sleep (insomnia)**: this may take the form of initial insomnia, broken sleep and/or early morning waking. The latter is the most significant diagnostically. Occasionally, depressed subjects (especially those with 'atypical' depression and/or seasonal affective disorder, SAD) report hypersomnia. Even when they do sleep, depressed patients characteristically complain of not feeling rested or refreshed on waking
  - **Fatigue/anergia**
  - **Poor appetite and weight loss**. As with sleep, some depressed patients

(e.g. those with SAD) report increased appetite (especially for carbohydrate-rich food) and weight gain
- **Diurnal variation of mood**: depressed patients typically report feeling worse first thing in the morning
- **Psychomotor retardation** or **agitation**: the latter is a very dangerous sign, since agitated patients are at high risk of self-harm, which they may attempt out of desperation
- **Dehydration and/or constipation**, especially in the elderly
- **Loss of libido**

- PSYCHOLOGICAL
  - Low mood
  - Anhedonia (inability to experience pleasure)
  - Self-blame and guilt
  - Feelings of hopelessness and pessimism about the future
  - Irritability
  - Suicidal ideation
- COGNITIVE
  - Poor concentration and increased distractibility
  - Memory impairment
  - Memory appears selective for 'unhappy' events
  - Negative self-appraisal/self-criticism

Depression may be accompanied by psychotic symptoms, the nature and content of which are almost always mood-congruent. They most commonly take the form of auditory hallucinations, often in the second person, and delusions, which typically have a negative or nihilistic content (e.g. that the patient's insides are rotting).

For a diagnosis of severe depression (ICD-10 F32.2) all three of the 'core' depressive symptoms must be present – i.e. depressed mood, loss of interest and enjoyment (anhedonia) and increased fatiguability – plus at least four other symptoms. A severe depressive episode should be of at least 2 weeks' duration.

EPIDEMIOLOGY

Manic-depressive psychosis

The lifetime risk of manic-depressive psychosis is about 0.5–1% in the general population. Prevalence of acute mania is about 0.5%. There are no clear sex or socioeconomic differences in prevalence or incidence of mania or manic-depressive psychosis. The first onset of mania/manic-depressive psychosis usually occurs before the age of 30 years, earlier than the onset of unipolar (non-psychotic) depression.

Unipolar depression

The prevalence of major depression is about 2–3% of the general population. The prevalence of moderate and mild depression is about 10–15%. Although less severe, mild depression accounts for about twice as many days of lost employment as major depression because of the higher prevalence.

The incidence of major depression is about 1–2% per year in the general population. The incidence of moderate and mild depression is about 5–10% per year.

The highest prevalence is in women (female:male, about 2:1). Recent evidence indicates that this is because of a higher incidence of depression among women rather than longer duration of individual episodes. Most evidence indicates that this sex difference is likely to be social in origin rather than the result of genetic differences or differences in sex hormones. There is some evidence that the sex difference in prevalence is greatest between the ages of 20 and 60 years, when the social roles of men and women are most clearly differentiated.

The prevalence is highest among those with the lowest socioeconomic status, although findings concerning occupational social class have been inconsistent. There is clear evidence that these disorders are strongly associated with measures of low material standard of living, including low income, living in rented accommodation and not having access to a car. Recent studies indicate that these associations are unlikely to be explained by social selection (i.e. downward social mobility).

Higher rates are also found in the unemployed, those with little or no education and those who are separated, divorced or widowed.

BASIC SCIENCE

Manic-depressive psychosis runs in families and there is evidence that this is the result of a genetic effect. Monozygotic/dizygotic concordance rates are about 4:1 (80% vs. 20%). The heritability of manic-depressive psychosis has been estimated to be 86%. Although there is no consistent evidence concerning specific genetic mechanisms, recent suggestions have included genes on chromosome 11 (reported in a large Amish family) and X-linked dominance with incomplete penetrance.

A genetic contribution has also been identified for unipolar major depression. A recent epidemiological twin study in the USA estimated that genetic factors accounted for 11% of the variance in liability to major depression, compared with recent life events (15%), past history of major depression (9%), neuroticism (6%), 'recent difficulties' (including financial hardship; 4%) and lack of parental warmth (4%).

While it has been shown consistently that threatening life events in the preceding 3 months are causally associated with the incidence of depression, there is also evidence that this association may be modified by material circumstances, occupational social class, self-esteem, childhood experiences and social support, particularly that elicited at times of crisis.

Theories concerning the mechanisms within the brain by which the symptoms of mania and depression arise have concentrated on noradrenaline (norepinephrine) and 5-HT (serotonin). According to the simplest version of the amine hypothesis, depressive symptoms are associated with low levels of noradrenaline and 5-HT, and manic symptoms with an excess of these transmitters.

While this hypothesis is partially supported by the finding of low levels of 3-methoxy-4-hydroxyphenylglycol (MHPG; a metabolite of noradrenaline) in the urine of depressed subjects, and low levels of 5-HT and 5-HT metabolites in suicides (post-mortem), there are also inconsistencies, including the unexplained delay in the onset of clinical response to antidepressants.

DIFFERENTIAL DIAGNOSIS OF MANIA

- **ORGANIC**
  - Frontal lobe syndromes associated with disinhibition, thought disorder, inappropriate affective responses and chaotic behaviour. Possible causes include tumours, infection, trauma and degenerative diseases such as Pick's disease
  - Drug-induced mania such as may be precipitated by steroids, amphetamines, cocaine and hallucinogens
  - Multiple sclerosis
  - Temporal lobe epilepsy
  - Wilson's disease
  - Hyperthyroidism
- **PSYCHIATRIC**

  Schizophrenia may be difficult to exclude in the presence of schneiderian first-rank symptoms. Important diagnostic features include family psychiatric history (i.e. tendency for different conditions to 'breed true'), past psychiatric history (although schizophrenia can also be associated with features of depression) and degree of symptomatic recovery between episodes. Note past controversy over concepts such as 'unitary psychosis' and 'schizoaffective disorders'

DIFFERENTIAL DIAGNOSIS OF DEPRESSION

- **ORGANIC**
  - Endocrine disorders: Cushing's disease, hypothyroidism, hyperparathyroidism
  - Drugs, including alcohol, corticosteroids, methyldopa, propranolol, cimetidine and amfetamine withdrawal
  - Head injury
  - Neoplasms, particularly carcinoma of the pancreas, brain and lung
  - Malnutrition, regardless of cause (including anorexia). May be mediated by vitamin B_{12} deficiency
  - Dementia, which may mimic depression (and vice versa)
  - Postviral fatigue, although the status of this diagnosis remains in doubt

  Note that with the exception of dementia, all the above represent organic *causes* of depression.
- **PSYCHIATRIC**
  - Schizophrenia

- Alcohol dependency syndrome
- Obsessive–compulsive disorder
- Generalized anxiety disorder

Note that all of these may either mimic depression or coexist with it as either a primary or secondary psychiatric condition. Indeed, it is extremely rare for depression to occur in the absence of significant anxiety.

MANAGEMENT OF AFFECTIVE DISORDERS

Management of mania

Acute management

Assess carefully and tactfully. Manic patients are often poor historians and are usually impatient, terminating interviews without warning. Always try to get an account of recent events from an informant. Beware irritability and quick temper – make sure backup is available. Most important information: any recent drug use, any current physical health problems, plus past psychiatric history and treatment. Does the patient normally take lithium? Important to ask about psychotic symptoms, plus understanding of current illness (insight) and willingness to accept treatment.

If not psychotic, willing to accept treatment, no danger to themselves or others and supported in the community, consider treating as an outpatient. In the short-term the best treatment is neuroleptic medication, e.g. chlorpromazine 100–200 mg daily. Patients who have stopped taking lithium recently should be strongly recommended to start taking it again. The main limitation of this approach is that manic patients characteristically lack insight, and compliance with medication is often inconsistent.

If psychotic, uncompliant, unsupported or judged to be dangerous (including risk of further deterioration in the patient's own health), admission is mandatory. Medication should be commenced at once. Neuroleptic medication may be augmented by benzodiazepines and/or lithium. Such patients will require intensive nursing care and may also need rapid tranquillization (see pp. 17–19) during the acute phase of their illness, especially as they may be very aroused by being forcibly detained in hospital.

Patients unresponsive to the above may benefit from electroconvulsive therapy.

Relapse prevention

The mainstay of relapse prevention is the prescription of mood-stabilizing drugs, i.e. lithium, carbamazepine and (less commonly) sodium valproate. Other drugs that are believed to act in this way are clonazepam and verapamil.

Patients with this disorder need counselling about the likely prognosis, the importance of maintaining compliance with their medication and 'early warning signs' indicative of relapse (such as initial insomnia). If such features can be identified it may be possible to formulate an 'emergency' strategy to be implemented in the case of relapse, since some patients retain insight in the prodromal stages of an acute episode of mania. Besides this supportive psychotherapy, recovered patients may also require considerable practical assistance in returning to the community, where they must repair any financial, physical and emotional damage done in the acute phase of their illness.

Although some centres attempt psychodynamic psychotherapy with patients with a history of manic-depressive psychosis, this type of intervention may precipitate manic relapses and a history of mania is generally viewed as a contraindication for this type of treatment.

Management of depression

Acute management

If psychotic and/or suicidal, the patient requires admission. The first priority in management is the patient's safety, and continuous nursing observation is mandatory. It is important to ask about current suicidal thoughts and plans, previous attempts at suicidal or deliberate self-harm and any family history of suicide. Agitated patients are at high risk of self-harm.

The first line of treatment in severe depression is a tricyclic antidepressant, unless contraindicated. The main contraindications are coexisting cardiac disease, including recent myocardial infarction or arrhythmias, and intolerance of anticholinergic side-effects (e.g. urinary retention). Among tricyclic drugs, the choice is between those that are more or less sedating. Amitriptyline and dothiepin (dosulepin) are much more sedating than imipramine, desipramine and lofepramine. In addition, lofepramine has a weaker anticholinergic effect and is far safer in overdose. (Note that it is not yet known at what level of severity of depression the benefits of such treatment outweigh the drawbacks.)

The main alternatives to tricyclic drugs are the SSRIs such as fluoxetine and sertraline, which do not have anticholinergic side-effects, are not sedating and are safe in overdose. There is no evidence that SSRIs are any more effective than tricyclics. The main side-effects of these drugs are nausea, diarrhoea and agitation. One advantage of starting with a tricyclic drug is that a drug-free interval of 1 week is required when changing from an SSRI to a tricyclic.

Neither class of antidepressant has an antidepressant effect for the first 10–14 days.

If the patient does not respond to 6 weeks of treatment on a therapeutic dose of a tricyclic (equivalent to 150 mg amitriptyline for 4 weeks) or an SSRI (e.g. fluoxetine 20 mg for 4 weeks), consider increasing the dose of current medication or changing to an antidepressant of a different class. If this fails, augmentation with lithium or L-thyronine may help. Little is known about the effects of combination treatment with a tricyclic and an SSRI.

Neuroleptic medication, such as risperidone, should be used if the depression is accompanied by psychotic symptoms. This drug is also very effective in treating any agitation, particularly among the elderly where this is a not infrequent feature.

Electroconvulsive therapy is indicated in the management of resistant depression and where antidepressants are contraindicated (e.g. some elderly patients), or when the patient's life may be at risk (from suicide or dehydration, arising from a refusal to eat or drink).

Psychological treatments: cognitive therapy (see pp. 240–241) appears to be as effective as antidepressant medication in treating the acute phase of moderate and severe depression.

Relapse prevention

Depression is a relapsing and remitting disorder, and those who have suffered even a single episode are at greatly increased risk of future episodes.

It is recommended that any antidepressant medication should be continued for a minimum of 6 months after the resolution of the acute episode.

Cognitive therapy appears to be superior to antidepressant treatment in preventing relapse. Some individuals who have suffered from depression may be suitable for individual or group psychodynamic psychotherapy. This type of treatment requires a significant investment of time (and sometimes money) on the part of the patient, and definitive evidence of clinical effectiveness has yet to be demonstrated.

NEUROTIC DISORDERS

Although psychiatrists traditionally subdivide the non-psychotic disorders into a series of distinct clinical entities, pure examples of these disorders are rare in community settings. Epidemiological evidence indicates that anxiety and depression are highly correlated and the majority of individuals suffering from these conditions experience both types of symptom (i.e. mixed anxiety/depression). Indeed, in primary-care and community settings, the most common disorder identified in epidemiological surveys is mixed anxiety depressive disorder (ICD-10 F41.2), perhaps the least satisfactory of all conditions from a nosological standpoint.

The more severe disorders are found most commonly in psychiatric settings, where it is often possible to distinguish among (primary) depression, generalized anxiety disorder, phobias, panic disorder and obsessive–compulsive disorder. All of neurotic disorders are characterized by the experience of anxiety to a greater or lesser degree.

CLINICAL FEATURES

Anxiety

- **IDEATIONAL**
  Fear and apprehension, particularly of 'losing control' over bodily functions
- **SOMATIC SYMPTOMS OF AUTONOMIC AROUSAL**
  Including dizziness, sweating, dry mouth, palpitations, choking, shortness of breath, hyperventilation, tremor, headache, backache, flushing, nausea, diarrhoea, urinary frequency. These symptoms may mimic cardiovascular disease, particularly if accompanied by chest pain. These symptoms may be exacerbated by hyperventilation and/or overbreathing, which may also result in dizziness, perioral and limb paraesthesias, and muscular spasm

- **PSYCHOLOGICAL**
  Hypervigilance, exaggerated startle response, irritability, sensitivity to noise, and rumination
- **BEHAVIOURAL**
  Avoidance of anxiety-provoking stimuli, leading to social isolation

Phobias

In phobic disorders, anxiety is evoked only (or predominantly) by well-defined situations or objects. The three most common phobias are agoraphobia, social phobia and simple phobia (ICD-10 F40), although the boundaries between these are often blurred. Phobias are often associated with panic attacks, which may be seen as an indicator of the severity of the phobia and/or the ubiquity of the phobic stimuli. Where panic attacks occur in the context of phobias, the latter are given diagnostic priority in ICD-10. In the case of agoraphobia, a further subclassification within ICD-10 allows the presence or absence of panic attacks to be coded.

- **AGORAPHOBIA**
  Excessive worry and anxiety about being away from home, and is usually worse in situations that do not permit immediate escape such as crowded shopping areas, lifts or public transport
- **SOCIAL PHOBIA**
  Intense fear of being scrutinized by other people, which usually manifests itself in a fear of performing even the most mundane of activities in front of others. Those with social phobia are most often afraid of eating in front of other people
- **SIMPLE PHOBIAS**
  Fears of very specific situations. Common stimuli are animals, insects, blood, dirt or contamination, heights and specific forms of travel (e.g. air travel). The latter may be difficult to distinguish from agoraphobia, although this distinction is probably of little clinical importance

Panic disorder

Panic disorder (F41.0) involves discrete periods of intense fear or apprehension in which several of the symptoms of anxiety (see above) develop *suddenly* and increase in intensity over about 10 minutes. Patients characteristically believe they are in imminent danger of 'losing control'; common fears are of collapsing, having a heart attack, 'going crazy' or being incontinent. Panic attacks tend to subside within 30 minutes and, characteristically, subjects do not experience anxiety between panic attacks. For diagnosis, the patient must have had several such attacks in 4 weeks and at least four somatic symptoms must be present during each attack. When panic attacks are associated with phobias, the latter are given diagnostic precedence in ICD-10.

Obsessive–compulsive disorder

Obsessions are repetitive, intrusive ideas, images and thoughts. Although unpleasant and unwanted, the subject feels that these are their own thoughts. The occurrence of obsessional thoughts is characteristically associated with an increase in anxiety, leading to rumination, rituals and compulsions, all of which may be viewed as means of reducing anxiety. Three-quarters of those with obsessional thoughts manifest compulsions, which frequently involve washing, cleaning and counting.

For a diagnosis of obsessive–compulsive disorder (OCD; ICD-10 F42), symptoms (obsessional thoughts and/or compulsions) must have been present on most days for at least 2 weeks; obsessional thoughts must be recognized as the subject's own; at least one thought or action must be resisted; the compulsion must not be pleasurable in itself (other than as a way of relieving anxiety); and the thoughts or compulsive acts must be unpleasantly repetitive.

Post-traumatic stress disorder

Post-traumatic stress disorder (PTSD; ICD-10 F43.1) arises, by definition, following the experience of a traumatic event beyond the range of 'normal' human experience, and usually involves the threat to, or loss of, life. PTSD is characterized by the persistent re-experience of the trauma, in the form of nightmares, 'flashbacks' and/or intrusive memories, often against a background sense of 'numbness' and detachment. Other features are depressed mood, anxiety, insomnia, poor concentration, irritability, hypervigilance, enhanced startle reaction and avoidance of situations that are reminiscent of the trauma. According to ICD-10, PTSD should not be diagnosed unless there is evidence that the condition arose within 6 months of a traumatic event.

The nosological status of PTSD remains controversial, particularly since it is the only psychiatric diagnosis included in ICD-10 to contain aetiological (as opposed to descriptive) criteria. Furthermore, PTSD may sometimes by seen by law courts as synonymous with a significant degree of emotional suffering following trauma.

SOMATOFORM DISORDERS

The classification of somatoform disorders within ICD-10 (F45) is complex. This probably reflects the aetiological uncertainty surrounding these conditions, persistence of the false dichotomy between psyche and soma, and continued belief within and without psychiatry about unconscious processes of 'conversion'. The evidence base in this area remains incomplete. These conditions, which are likely to be multifactorial in origin, are best viewed under the general rubric of 'abnormal illness behaviour'. As this implies, it is increasingly recognized that the quantity and quality of an individual's interactions with medical services is often inappropriate in these conditions. Broadly, those suffering from somatoform disorders may be differentiated according to whether they are convinced that they are suffering from a physical illness (somatization), or morbidly afraid that this is the case (hypochondriasis). In addition, some of the dissociative disorders (F44) also present with alterations in physical functioning, coupled with persistent medical help-seeking, and may be considered as abnormal illness behaviour.

Somatization disorder

Somatization disorder is characterized by multiple (and often changing) unexplained somatic complaints, typically affecting several different organ systems, for which an individual repeatedly seeks medical care. Such individuals will often request investigations or specialist referrals, despite the absence of evidence of a physical basis for their complaints. Negative test results and repeated reassurance from doctors rarely brings either psychological or physical relief and the pursuit of further investigation is often relentless. It is common for patients to change doctors frequently in this quest. A number of names have been coined for this group of individuals, including 'heartsink patient' and 'fat-folder patient'. Most such individuals will strongly resist discussion of psychosocial or emotional difficulties, even when it is clear that these are linked with the onset or exacerbation of their symptoms.

For a formal diagnosis of somatization disorder, ICD-10 (F45.0) requires that multiple unexplained physical symptoms should have been present for at least 2 years, that the patient should refuse to accept reassurance from several doctors that there is no physical explanation for their symptoms; and that there should be significant social impairment arising from these complaints.

Hypochondriacal disorder

The main feature of this condition (ICD-10 F45.2) is a morbid preoccupation with, and fear of, serious (physical) disease. As in patients with somatization disorder, it is believed that an important underlying mechanism for this condition is a tendency to misinterpret normal physiological sensations. However, unlike patients with somatization disorder, who are convinced that they are ill and who want treatment, hypochondriacal patients are terrified that they might be ill and would prefer to avoid treatment. Marked depression and anxiety are often present, and will usually be acknowledged, at least as a secondary source of distress.

Hypochondriasis may be viewed primarily as an anxiety disorder and shares many common features with obsessive–compulsive disorder. One particularly troubling form of hypochondriacal disorder is body dysmorphic disorder, in which sufferers develop obsessional and extremely disabling thoughts about (usually) one specific aspect of their appearance, such as the shape of their nose.

EPIDEMIOLOGY

In the UK, the overall prevalence of non-psychotic psychiatric disorder in the community is approximately 16%. The most common ICD-10 diagnosis is mixed anxiety and depressive disorder, identified in nearly 8% of adults living in private households (in 1991). About 2% of adults suffer from severe or moderately severe depression, and 3% from generalized anxiety disorder. About 5–6% of adults suffer from the other neurotic disorders – phobias, panic disorder and obsessive–compulsive disorder – each of which has a prevalence of about 1–2%. There are no good epidemiological studies of the prevalence or incidence of PTSD or the somatoform disorders.

The non-psychotic psychiatric disorders (particularly anxiety and depression) are strongly associated with indices of low socioeconomic status, such as unemployment, low income, poor housing and financial hardship. Collectively, these disorders are more common among women than men, with a gender difference in the prevalence of depression of between 1.5 and 2 across all community settings and using a range of different measures. The explanation for this remains obscure but it is not caused by differences in help-seeking or diagnostic practice. Although higher rates of these disorders have been reported in some ethnic groups in the UK (such as south Asians), the epidemiological evidence base in this area remains weak. Recent research has tended to disprove simplistic notions about differences in the frequency and manner of medical help-seeking among individuals from different cultural and ethnic backgrounds. In particular, the notion that some ethnic and cultural groups are more likely to 'somatize' emotional distress is no longer current.

BASIC SCIENCES

There is evidence of a significant genetic contribution to the aetiology of the non-psychotic disorders, including depression, generalized anxiety and panic disorder. A consensus now exists that genes account for about 30–40% of the variance in symptoms of anxiety and depression, as well the occurrence of the most common ICD-10 disorders, including depressive episodes, generalized anxiety disorder and the phobias. There is also evidence that the genetic risk is common to all of these, and is not condition-specific.

Positron emission tomography scanning studies have shown increased cerebral metabolic activity in the cingulate region and heads of the caudate nuclei and orbital gyri in individuals with obsessive–compulsive disorder, as well as with related conditions such as Tourette's syndrome. It is not clear, however, whether obsessional thoughts are caused directly by this abnormal activity or whether they arise indirectly, because of a failure of this dysfunctional area of cortex to filter out such thoughts. There is also evidence that OCD is associated with a relative deficiency of 5-HT, since this condition responds to SSRIs (see pp. 225–228).

Environmental factors are likely to be of aetiological importance, although the extent to which such circumstances are determined genetically remains unclear. The clearest example of the importance of environmental influences in the pathogenesis of the neurotic disorders can be seen in post-traumatic stress disorder, which can only arise following the experience of a severe trauma. Onset of PTSD may be delayed for several months, and the incidence among those exposed would appear to depend on subjects' premorbid characteristics and the severity of the trauma. This model of the pathogenesis of PTSD is consistent with extensive research documenting a causal association between threatening life events and the onset of both anxiety and depression. There is some evidence that the type of event encountered may by pathoplastic, in that anxiety is reported to follow events characterized by danger, while the onset of depression is more closely associated with events characterized by loss. However, most epidemiological research indicates that the risk associated with environmental factors is only marginally more condition-specific than the genetic risk, which appears to be common to all non-psychotic disorders.

DIFFERENTIAL DIAGNOSIS OF ANXIETY

ORGANIC

- Alcohol or drug withdrawal/intoxication, including delirium tremens, may produce restlessness, agitation, poor concentration and subjective anxiety, apprehension or fearfulness. Anxiety and neurotic disorders are *not* associated with disorientation or fluctuations in level of consciousness. Enquire about drug and alcohol use and look for signs of this. Drugs can be detected by testing urine, and liver function tests may be abnormal. Remember that anxious people may self-medicate with alcohol or drugs, and try to elucidate the primary pathology by means of careful history-taking
- Thyrotoxicosis causes sweating, tachycardia, tremor and agitation. Look for signs of thyroid disease, including goitre and ophthalmic complications
- Hypoglycaemia may present with symptoms of anxiety, although onset will be acute and the subject should be symptom-free except when hypoglycaemic. Enquire about history of diabetes and check random blood glucose
- In both phaeochromocytoma and carcinoid syndrome, both of which are extremely rare, anxiety, sweating, agitation, headaches and hypertension are episodic. It is possible to test urine for vanillylmandelic acid and 5-HIAA following 24-hour collection
- Angina/cardiac arrhythmias may present with palpitations, chest pain, and shortness of breath

PSYCHIATRIC

- Schizophrenia may mimic OCD. Remember that in OCD unwanted experiences are almost always perceived as arising from the subject's own mind. In OCD, patients will admit to finding it difficult to resist intrusive thoughts or compulsive behaviours but will not usually describe these as being controlled by outside agencies
- Mania
- Other neurotic disorder, including depression
- Dementia (see pp. 202–205)
- Personality disorder, although this should only be considered as a diagnosis of last resort

- Hyperventilation syndrome, a 'condition' in which individuals over-breathe and then experience the somatic symptoms associated with hyperventilation (e.g. paraesthesias). Classically, these symptoms then induce high levels of anxiety in turn, positively reinforcing this behaviour

MANAGEMENT

- Although neurotic disorder is common in the community, referral to psychiatrists is rare. Most treatment is therefore provided by GPs, particularly for the more common (and less severe) disorders. In the case of mixed anxiety and depressive disorder, there is little empirical evidence to guide treatment and it is not known at what threshold of severity individuals benefit from antidepressant medication, or what the optimum dose of this should be. Similarly, it is not known whether such individuals might derive greater benefit from psychological than pharmacological interventions or whether (for example) seeing a social worker is more effective than problem-solving, cognitive behavioural therapy or psychoeducation
- More is known, however, about the treatment of the more severe anxiety disorders seen in psychiatric settings, for which first-line management usually involves behavioural and/or cognitive psychotherapy (see pp. 234–244). Behavioural psychotherapy for the anxiety disorders is based on the concept of cue exposure and response prevention. The role of the therapist is to help the patient identify a graded hierarchy of fear-inducing situations and to overcome each of these in order, beginning with the least threatening. In most cases, cue exposure begins with the patient imagining or talking about the anxiety-provoking situation. The main goal of therapy is for the patient to tolerate exposure to the stimulus while resisting the urge to engage in avoidant or explicitly anxiety-reducing behaviours (such as compulsions or rituals) for which they have sought treatment. It is necessary to explain to the patient that anxiety is a universal human experience, that intense anxiety can be tolerated without adverse effects and that doing so will reduce both the future frequency and intensity of anxiety attacks. Such therapy may be successfully augmented by the use of relaxation techniques
- Although limited use of a benzodiazepine (alprazolam) is recommended (especially in the USA), evidence indicates that this is no more effective than behavioural psychotherapy alone. While alprazolam alone may be as effective as behavioural psychotherapy initially, relapse occurs almost as soon as the medication is discontinued. Long-term benzodiazepine use is associated with dependence and a recognized withdrawal syndrome. Caution is recommended in the prescription of benzodiazepines
- The use of antidepressants (especially SSRIs) may be helpful, although to date there is no evidence to indicate whether combining these with psychological treatment is better than either treatment on its own. While the benefit of antidepressants is clear-cut where features of depression occur, there is also evidence that SSRIs may have a beneficial effect even in their absence. Evidence indicates, however, that the anxiolytic effects of SSRIs

(such as paroxetine and sertraline) may be most marked at doses higher than those commonly used for the treatment of depression. It is also important to be aware that some of these drugs (especially fluoxetine) may cause agitation and restlessness, especially in the early stages of treatment

EATING DISORDERS I: ANOREXIA NERVOSA

CLINICAL FEATURES

Anorexia nervosa (ICD-10 F50.0) is characterized by self-induced weight loss, resulting in a body mass index (BMI) below 17.5, accompanied by a fear of fatness and endocrine disorders (amenorrhoea in females, loss of libido and sexual dysfunction in men).

BMI = weight (kg)/height (m)^2; the normal range for BMI is 20–25.

Behavioural

Weight loss may be achieved by avoidance of food, excessive exercise and/or the use of appetite suppressants, laxatives and diuretics. Patients may describe subjective binges (usually of smaller quantities of food than described by patients with bulimia nervosa), and self-induced vomiting may also be a feature. It is the presence of low weight that confirms the diagnosis of anorexia nervosa.

Physical

Patients with anorexia may recognize some of the effects of low weight, which include dry skin, poor condition of nails and hair, tiredness, sensitivity to the cold, dizziness, constipation, lack of libido, amenorrhoea in females and sexual dysfunction in males. They are less likely to recognize that they are underweight and tend to conceal their bodies with loose-fitting clothing, fearing that they are overweight. Physical complications are secondary to malnutrition and include the following.

- **CARDIOVASCULAR**
  Bradycardia (HR <60), hypotension (BP 90/60) ventricular arrhythmias and/or cardiac failure. Marked postural hypotension is evidence of dehydration. Reversible ECG abnormalities including prolonged QT or QTc interval, which may be an indicator of an increased risk of sudden death from arrhythmias. Tachycardia may indicate an underlying infection

- **METABOLIC**
  Hypothermia, hypoglycaemia and hypercholesterolaemia. Diuretic abuse and/or vomiting may cause hypokalaemia and altered blood pH

- **GASTROINTESTINAL**
  Constipation and diarrhoea are common. Diarrhoea may be due to laxative abuse or irritable bowel syndrome, which is common in patients with anorexia nervosa. Starvation leads to fatty changes in liver and hepatomegaly. Acute pancreatitis can occur on refeeding
- **RENAL**
  Renal calculi, resulting from altered pH balance and dehydration, low glomerular filtration rate and low serum magnesium; may also lead to renal failure
- **HAEMATOLOGICAL**
  Pancytopenia, anaemia and bone marrow hypoplasia
- **ENDOCRINE**
  Disturbance of sex hormone metabolism, low luteinizing hormone (LH) and follicle-stimulating hormone (FSH) in women and low testosterone in men, impaired oogenesis and spermatogenesis, stress hormones elevated, including growth hormone and cortisol. This disturbance of the hypothalamic–pituitary–gonadal axis is responsible for amenorrhoea in women and loss of libido in men
- **MUSCULOSKELETAL**
  Osteoporosis and/or retarded bony maturation, proximal myopathy
- **NEUROLOGICAL**
  Seizures

Psychological

Sufferers frequently experience a distorted body image, believing themselves to be larger (and fatter) than they are, although this is no longer considered a necessary criteria for anorexia nervosa. Anorexia nervosa is characterized by a rigid, obsessional preoccupation with food, body weight and physical appearance. Patients with anorexia nervosa may resemble sufferers of OCD in their dread of losing control over their weight.

As a result of starvation, sleep may become disturbed, with shortened REM latency, and mood may become depressed, with irritability, anhedonia, hopelessness and suicidal thoughts.

Social

Poor concentration and fatigue may lead to difficulty coping and time off work. Sufferers may withdraw from social contact because of feelings of worthlessness associated with their body image, and because they feel less able to engage in conversation while preoccupied with food. Anxiety and concern expressed by family members about eating behaviour may lead to conflict with loved ones, increasing the sense of isolation and loneliness.

EPIDEMIOLOGY

The annual incidence of anorexia nervosa is approximately 7:100 000 population. The median age of onset is 17 but the age range is 8–60 years. Over 90% of cases occur in women. The recorded prevalence among young women (age 15–29 years) in general practice is about 0.15%. Particularly high rates of anorexia are reported among ballet dancers and models (6–7%) and in middle and upper socioeconomic groups. The median duration of illness is 5–6 years, with a third of cases having a more chronic course. Anorexia nervosa has the highest mortality of any psychiatric illness, with an SMR five times higher than expected. The mortality rate is approximately 1% per year, with approximately 50% of deaths due to medical complications and 50% resulting from suicide.

BASIC SCIENCES

Abnormalities in the hypothalamic–pituitary–gonadal axis and the hypothalamic–pituitary–adrenal axis are present, resulting in increased cortisol secretion with loss of diurnal variation and dexamethasone suppression, increased growth hormone, decreased LH, FSH, oestrogen, thyroid-stimulating hormone (TSH) and triiodothyronine. These abnormalities have been replicated in previously healthy subjects under conditions of starvation and normalize with refeeding, suggesting that these abnormalities in anorexia nervosa are not causal. Genetic studies indicate that monozygotic concordance is significantly higher than dizygotic concordance.

Social explanations for anorexia point to the culture-specific nature of anorexia nervosa, which is less common in developing countries. Most attention has been directed towards the fashion industry in Western societies and the intense social pressure for young women to aspire and conform to one particular image of female beauty. Psychodynamic theories propose that the delayed puberty of amenorrhoea is an expression of a subconscious desire to avoid (or at least to control) the emergence of an adult female sexual identity. The model of the psychosomatic family developed by Minuchin is that of a family characterized by enmeshment, rigidity and over-protectiveness, where the illness of a physiologically vulnerable child has the function of enabling conflict avoidance. A severe life event precedes the onset of anorexia nervosa in three-quarters of cases. A multifactorial model of anorexia nervosa would therefore be that of a genetically determined abnormality of appetite regulation, triggered under conditions of stress and maintained by family and social factors.

DIFFERENTIAL DIAGNOSIS

ORGANIC

- Hypopituitarism (note that in anorexia nervosa axillary and pubic hair, if established, remain intact)
- Addison's disease (in cases of pituitary disturbance consider a space-occupying lesion)

- Thyrotoxicosis
- Inflammatory bowel disease/malabsorption (e.g. Crohn's disease or coeliac disease)
- Diabetes mellitus
- Carcinoma
- Infection (especially tuberculosis and HIV)

PSYCHIATRIC

- Bulimia nervosa
- Depression
- Obsessive–compulsive disorder, which is also characterized by intrusive, unwanted, repetitive, anxiety-provoking thoughts. It has been suggested that anorexia is a variant of OCD, on the basis that sufferers commonly have obsessional traits that predate the illness and that OCD is more common in the mothers of anorexic patients. It is possible that both may be mediated by abnormalities in 5-HT transmission

MANAGEMENT

- The main aim of treatment is the restoration of a healthy weight and healthy eating habits. This is best achieved gradually, and success depends on the establishment of a therapeutic alliance with the patient. Patients often come for assessment at the insistence of concerned relatives and are likely to be highly ambivalent about the aim of weight gain. Attempts to persuade or confront the patient are generally counterproductive, as the patient fears a loss of control over their body and responds with a more determined refusal of the help offered. Motivational interviewing offers an approach that collaboratively explores the ambivalence to change and the possible outcomes, with a view to helping the patient make an informed choice about whether to engage in further treatment with the aim of weight gain. The majority of patients can be treated with outpatient psychotherapy combined with weight monitoring and dietary advice. Antidepressants are ineffective in patients with a low body weight and should be discontinued because of the risk of side-effects. Younger patients living at home may respond to family therapy. Day hospital or inpatient treatment on a specialist unit is appropriate where previous outpatient therapy has failed, where there is social isolation or an intolerable family situation
- Urgent hospital admission to a specialist unit should be considered in the presence of the following signs, which indicate an increased risk of physical mortality due to starvation:
  - If weight loss is severe (BMI <13.5), especially if more than 25% of body weight has been lost in the past 6 months
  - Signs of marrow failure (e.g. petechial haemorrhages)
  - Hypoglycaemia
  - Severe electrolyte disturbance (e.g. hypokalaemia, $K < 2.5$)
  - Circulatory failure (pulse <45, BP $<70/60$, frequent faints), or a prolonged QT interval on ECG

  - Proximal myopathy (a simple test is to ask the patient to rise from a squatting position without assistance)
- Inpatient treatment should be provided in a specialist unit wherever possible because of evidence of improved outcomes. Weight restoration is largely through regular mealtimes in a ward milieu that is structured with clear rules. Meals should be supervised by nurses who eat with the group, encouraging peer support and challenging anorexic behaviour. Weight gain should be gradual at first to reduce patient anxiety and the risk of potential physical complications. A soft diet is provided initially and then increased to provide approximately 3000 kcal/day and a weight gain of 1–2 kg a week. A target weight range is provided for the patient, usually based on their weight prior to their illness. Patients may develop rebound oedema on refeeding; less common complications include acute gastric dilatation and hypophosphataemia
- Compulsory treatment can be provided under the Mental Health Act 1983, which includes refeeding within its definition of nursing care. On a specialized unit, nasogastric feeding should only be necessary in rare cases (1%). A multidisciplinary approach is important and should include the provision of individual and group therapy, family counselling, dietary advice, occupational therapy and rehabilitation

EATING DISORDERS II: BULIMIA NERVOSA

CLINICAL FEATURES

Bulimia nervosa (ICD-10 F50.2) is characterized by repeated binge eating associated with recurrent compensatory behaviour to avoid weight gain (e.g. self-induced vomiting, laxative abuse and excessive exercise). As in anorexia, those suffering from bulimia nervosa are often preoccupied with their weight and appearance. In contrast to anorexia nervosa, patients with bulimia nervosa are of normal, or slightly above-normal weight. If symptoms of bulimia occur in association with those of anorexia nervosa, the latter is given diagnostic primacy (note that DSM-IV includes a category of anorexia nervosa, binge/purge subtype). Although ICD-10 does not define the frequency of bingeing and purging behaviour required, DSM-IV requires that one or other of these occur at least twice a week for 3 months for a diagnosis of bulimia nervosa.

Binge eating is defined as the consumption of a clearly excessive amount of food within a discrete period (2 hours), associated with a sense of loss of control. Purging often immediately follows a binge and is usually in the form of self-induced vomiting. Patients may have restricted their food for hours or days prior to a binge and often experience an intense craving for food.

Episodes of bingeing and purging may be precipitated by feelings of depression, anxiety, boredom or loneliness. Foods selected for binges may be those that the individual perceives as forbidden (e.g. chocolate bars, cakes and biscuits) and that they usually deny themselves. As many as 10 000 kcal may be consumed in a single episode, which is usually followed by feelings of intense guilt, shame and self-loathing. The time and financial cost of supplying food for severe and frequent binges can be considerable.

Depression is more common in patients with bulimia nervosa than in those with anorexia, and 30–50% meet the criteria for major depression. Comorbid personality disorder is also common, and bulimic symptoms may occur as one of a variety of impulsive, self harming behaviours in patients with borderline personality disorder. Bulimic behaviour may develop in up to 30% of patients recovering from anorexia nervosa.

The physical sequelae of bulimia are mainly secondary to the purging behaviour, and the most common are:

- Parotid gland enlargement, leading to the appearance of puffy cheeks
- Erosion of dental enamel
- Calluses on the dorsum of the hand (Russell's sign)
- Metabolic disturbances, especially alkalosis and hypokalaemia.

EPIDEMIOLOGY

Bulimia nervosa was first described by Russell in 1979. Rates of presentation in primary-care settings increased threefold between 1988 and 1993, possibly as a result of increased public and medical awareness of the condition. Bulimic symptoms are fairly common but the fluctuating course and problems of definition make epidemiological precision difficult. The current annual incidence of presentation in primary care is thought to be 10–13:100 000 population. The community prevalence is approximately 1–3%, of whom 90% are female.

BASIC SCIENCE

Although most studies show an increased concordance for monozygotic compared to dizygotic twins, this concordance is less marked than for patients with anorexia nervosa, suggesting that genetic factors may be less important. Patients with bulimia are more likely than controls to come from a family with a history of obesity, or where there is a preoccupation with food. Severe life events precede the onset of bulimia nervosa in 70% of cases. Bulimic patients are more likely than those with anorexia to have experienced abuse, neglect, parental discord or inconsistency in care arrangements. In common with anorexia, social influences in Western culture that encourage young women to focus on dieting behaviour as a means to improve their self-image are likely to reinforce bulimic behaviour. Central monoamine pathways, particularly of 5-HT, are thought to have an inhibitory effect on feeding behaviour and satiety mechanisms, and several studies have shown lowered central 5-HT in bulimic women. However, as with anorexia nervosa, interpretation is complicated by the possibility that dieting behaviour may contribute to these neurochemical abnormalities.

DIFFERENTIAL DIAGNOSIS

- **Upper gastrointestinal disorders, which cause repeated vomiting, e.g. duodenal ulcer**
- **Depression**
- **Personality disorder, particularly borderline type (ICD-10 F60.31)**

MANAGEMENT

- Cognitive behavioural therapy is the mainstay of treatment. A stepped approach to treatment is recommended, in which self-help manuals are used as a first measure (effective for 20% of patients), followed by individual or group psychotherapy for those who do not respond. Key elements in cognitive behavioural therapy for bulimia include
  - Keeping a diary of bingeing/purging behaviour, thoughts and feelings
  - Identifying triggers and devising strategies to reduce bulimic behaviour
  - Psychoeducation about how the cycle of dieting and bingeing/purging behaviour is self-perpetuating
  - Planning regular small meals and snacks (prolonged periods without food increase the risk of succumbing to a binge)

  Underlying basic assumptions (which often include low self worth) should be identified and alternative evidence examined
- The majority of patients can be managed as outpatients. Admission may be indicated, however, if the patient is severely depressed, at risk of suicide or if they are suffering from severe physical complications and have not responded to outpatient treatment. Some patients may, however, get worse in this setting and an initial brief admission for assessment may be appropriate
- Fluoxetine, at doses (60 mg daily) above those usually used in the treatment of depression, has been shown to be effective in reducing bulimic and depressive symptoms in patients with bulimia nervosa. Drug treatment appears to be less effective than cognitive behaviour therapy, which produces more substantial and long-lasting change, although antidepressants may be useful supplements to psychotherapy

DISORDERS OF PERSONALITY

The concept of personality disorder as a diagnostic entity has arisen out of attempts to classify a variety of dysfunctional behaviours that are often poorly understood and that are largely unresponsive to treatment. While psychologists have preferred to conceptualize personality in terms of a variety of continuously distributed traits, psychiatrists have traditionally opted instead for categorical models. Personality disorders therefore represent persistent and characteristic patterns of behaviour and ways of relating to the self and others. Central to the definition of personality disorder is the notion that these behaviours are harmful to the individual or others.

CLINICAL FEATURES

Personality disorders involve enduring maladaptive patterns of behaviour, modes of thinking and relating to oneself, the environment and others that cause either impairment in social functioning or considerable distress to the individual or others. These personality features should be recognizable by adolescence and should persist throughout adult life. Central to the concept of personality disorder within ICD-10 (F60–69) is the persistence of problematic behaviours across numerous settings and over time.

Personality disorders are primary and not secondary to other psychiatric or physical disorders.

Within ICD-10, personality disorders correspond to clusters of traits. A diagnosis of personality disorder should only be made on the basis of more than one interview with the patient, and with information from as many informants as possible. Eight specific personality disorders are listed in ICD-10.

Paranoid personality disorder (F60.0)

This involves excessive sensitivity to setbacks, a tendency to bear grudges and harbour resentments, suspiciousness, unwillingness to trust others, litigiousness and a preoccupation with 'conspiracy theories'. Individuals with paranoid personality disorder often suspect their spouse or partner of being unfaithful, and have a tendency towards self-importance. Such individuals are extremely 'brittle' and, contrary to their protestations, have an extremely fragile self-esteem, which they need to bolster continuously by means of projection.

Schizoid personality disorder (F60.1)

Cold and aloof, these individuals do not appear to take pleasure from any activities and seem incapable of expressing strong positive or negative emotions. Affect is cold, detached or flat. Such people have little capacity for, or interest in, intimate relationships (including sexual relationships). Thus, individuals with schizoid personality disorder have few friends and appear to prefer solitary pursuits. Social awkwardness may be very prominent. A further defining characteristic is an apparent insensitivity to praise or criticism.

Dissocial personality disorder (F60.2)

This is perhaps the most dangerous of all the personality disorders, characterized by antisocial behaviour and callous disregard for the feelings, safety and wellbeing of others. Dissocial personality disorder incorporates the earlier categories of sociopathic and psychopathic personality disorders. Those with dissocial personality disorder are irresponsible, show no concern for rules or social norms, and are often in conflict with authority. There is a characteristic inability to tolerate frustration, resulting in aggressive and violent behaviour. Individuals with dissocial personality disorder appear incapable of experiencing remorse and tend to blame others (including their victims) for their own shortcomings and misdeeds. There is some empirical evidence that such individuals are incapable of learning from punishment or reward, which may reflect underlying brain dysfunction.

Emotionally unstable personality disorder (F60.3)

Two types of emotionally unstable personality disorder are listed in ICD-10, **impulsive type** (F60.30) and **borderline type** (F60.31). Both are characterized by emotional instability, poor self-control and impulsive behaviour. Emotions are experienced with unbearable intensity, leading to explosive outbursts and/or attempts at self-harm. In the impulsive form of this personality disorder, individuals respond to criticism with violent or threatening outbursts. Individuals with borderline personality disorder are said to have a 'chronic sense of emptiness', and may become involved in intense and unstable personal relationships. Emotional crises are common, often arising out of a fear of abandonment. Such individuals may experience transient psychotic episodes, such is the intensity of their emotions. Some individuals with borderline personality disorder cope with their unbearable internal feelings by indulging in self-mutilating behaviours, such as cutting or burning their arms or legs, while others may take overdoses or make more serious attempts at suicide. The cardinal feature of self-mutilating behaviour in borderline personality disorder is that the patient reports an immediate release of anxiety on inflicting the wound (or on seeing their own blood).

Depression and eating disorders (anorexia and bulimia nervosa) are common among individuals with emotionally unstable personality disorder.

Histrionic personality disorder (F60.4)

This involves self-dramatizing and theatrical behaviour, often perceived by others as attention-seeking. There is a shallow, labile affect. Individuals with histrionic personality disorder seek excitement and gain a reputation for melodrama. They appear vain, egotistical and self-absorbed and are largely incapable of forming enduring close relationships or showing genuine concern for others. A characteristic scenario is that in which the support of friends or family is enlisted in dealing with a crisis that never materializes or that turns out to be rather trivial. The individual with histrionic personality disorder then moves on to the next 'crisis' without apparent concern for the distress this may cause others. As a result such individuals often alienate those nearest to them, gaining a reputation for 'crying wolf'.

Anankastic personality disorder (F60.5)

Characterized by caution, anxiety and self-doubt, such individuals are often described as 'obsessional', appearing preoccupied with order and the observation of rules. They are the archetypal 'perfectionists', a trait that ceases to be of benefit to the individual but instead leads to a paralysing rigidity in their approach to any task. The same applies to tidiness, conscientiousness, and scrupulousness: although assets in moderation, these traits are extremely damaging in their extreme forms. The anankastic individual is therefore pedantic and stubborn to an extent that precludes compromise or the formation of close relationships with others.

Anxious (avoidant) personality disorder (F60.6)

This is characterized by constant feelings of apprehension and low self-esteem, exacerbated by fear of social inadequacy. People with this type of personality disorder frequently consider themselves to be socially inept and unappealing to others. Fear of humiliation or rejection in social interactions leads to avoidance of other people. There is also hypersensitivity to, and fear of, criticism. There is a high degree of diagnostic overlap (comorbidity) between avoidant personality disorder and social phobia.

Dependent personality disorder (F60.7)

Such individuals are unwilling to take responsibility for important decisions in their lives, preferring for others to make them. Passivity and acquiescence with those on whom they depend is characteristic, as are feelings of helplessness when alone. Dependent individuals require enormous reassurance to make even the simplest independent decisions.

EPIDEMIOLOGY

There have been very few community-based epidemiological studies into personality disorders, in part because of the difficulty of defining, operationalizing and assessing the presence of these conditions. Studies of dissocial personality disorder indicate that the prevalence in the community is about 2–3%, rising to 60% in studies of male prisoners. Dissocial personality disorder has been found to be consistently more prevalent among men than women, across different settings. The prevalence of other personality disorders remains unknown. High rates of comorbidity have been documented between personality disorders (especially of the dissocial and emotionally unstable types) and drug and alcohol misuse, and depression. Personality disorder is also thought to represent an important risk factor for deliberate self-harm and suicide among depressed adults of all ages. Comorbidity has also been noted between anxiety disorders and certain types of personality disorder (cluster C, see below), although this is thought to be less commonplace than the comorbidity observed with depression.

Personality disorders are likely to be much more common in psychiatric settings than in the community. One review estimated that 20–50% of psychiatric inpatients and more than 50% of outpatients met diagnostic criteria for at least one personality disorder.

Previous studies have shown a high degree of comorbidity (i.e. diagnostic overlap) between the different types of personality disorder described in ICD-10 (and DSM-IV). There is evidence that personality disorders may be more validly represented by a three-cluster model (A, B and C) than by eight discrete categories. These clusters are as follows:

- **CLUSTER A**
  - Paranoid
  - Schizoid
- **CLUSTER B**
  - Dissocial
  - Emotionally unstable
  - Histrionic
- **CLUSTER C**
  - Anxious
  - Anankastic
  - Dependent

BASIC SCIENCE

Most aetiological enquiry in the field of personality disorders has focused on dissocial personality disorder (formerly referred to as psychopathy), a syndrome that rarely occurs in the absence of a history of childhood antisocial behaviour. Such individuals often come from disturbed homes, and associations have been reported with a paternal history of antisocial behaviour as well as with childhood physical and/or sexual abuse. Such findings are consistent with both biological (genetic) and environmental models.

Genetic studies have estimated concordance rates in dissocial personality disorder for monozygotic twins at 36% and for dizygotic twins at 12%, suggesting a strong genetic contribution.

There is also evidence of abnormal brain function among individuals with dissocial personality disorder. One well-known finding is that widespread slow waves are seen on the EEGs of up to 60% of individuals with this diagnosis. This neurophysiological abnormality appears to be more common among those with a history of aggressive or violent behaviour. It has been suggested that the inability to learn from noxious experiences (e.g. punishment) reflects cortical immaturity or minimal brain damage. The frontal and temporal lobes appear to be the most likely site of any focal abnormality.

Research has indicated strong associations between childhood abuse and emotionally unstable personality disorder.

DIFFERENTIAL DIAGNOSIS

The differential diagnosis will vary for different specific personality disorders. Although other psychiatric disorders can occur in the context of an abnormal or dysfunctional personality, it is usual to diagnose a personality disorder only in the absence of an alternative psychiatric diagnosis. In view of the stigma attached to 'personality disorder', this diagnosis should be made with extreme caution.

Thus, other major psychiatric disorders should be excluded before a diagnosis of personality disorder is made. The following should be considered:

- Schizophrenia (note that the negative symptoms of chronic schizophrenia can appear as apathy, passivity or dependence)
- Mania can mimic histrionic personality disorder
- Depression
- Generalized anxiety disorder/panic disorder/social phobia
- Obsessive–compulsive disorder
- Somatoform/dissociative disorders
- Drug and/or alcohol dependency
- Anorexia nervosa or bulimia nervosa

MANAGEMENT

- Since the defining feature of personality disorders is that they represent 'enduring maladaptive patterns of behaviour', prognosis is usually poor. It is therefore essential that treatment of such individuals is pragmatic. In general there is little likelihood of significant change in personality, although over longer periods of time dysfunctional behaviours may be modifiable. Few individuals with personality disorder enter into psychiatric treatment, and those that do are likely to be referred because of antisocial behaviour or severe difficulties in social functioning
- It is important to identify and treat any (other) psychiatric disorders, especially depression, or drug or alcohol dependency, which may exacerbate the expression of the comorbid personality disorder
- The dysfunctional behaviours that cause so much distress reflect interactions between the individual with personality disorder and his or her environment. Since personality is likely to be resistant to change, it is often much more productive and helpful to identify aspects of the patient's environment that might be modified. Thus, individuals with personality disorder can be advised to structure their lives (e.g. accommodation, occupation and social contacts) in such a way as to minimize conflict and psychological distress. Thus, the mainstay of treatment for most individuals with personality disorders is low-intensity supportive psychotherapy, combined with supervision of those individuals at risk of antisocial behaviour. An example of this might be advising the individual with paranoid personality disorder not to apply for a job that will involve working in an open-plan office
- Although it has been suggested that some patients with personality disorder may benefit from long-term psychoanalytic psychotherapy, there is little empirical evidence to support the effectiveness of such treatment
- The Mental Health Act 1983 makes provision for the formal (compulsory) treatment of just one type of personality disorder, the dissocial type. Although most psychiatrists believe such individuals to be resistant to treatment, this aspect of the Mental Health Act allows for individuals with dissocial personality disorder to be detained in psychiatric hospital (e.g. special hospitals) for the protection of others. This has recently become a

highly contentious issue, with most psychiatrists opposed to proposed changes to the Act that will require all those who are judged to be dangerous but who have not committed a crime to be detained in this way

OTHER BEHAVIOURAL DISORDERS

PUERPERAL DISORDERS

Although listed under this section within the ICD-10 classification, these disorders are discussed on pp. 83–86.

PSYCHOSEXUAL PROBLEMS

Sexual problems among the mentally ill have gained greater attention in recent years for several reasons.

- The mentally ill, despite disabilities, do have active sex lives and it is very stigmatizing for professionals to assume otherwise
- Mental illness and sexual functioning have several interfaces: for example, a confiding relationship may be a protective factor for depression and other disorders; expressed emotions invariably arise in the context of a relationship, of which sexual matters are one aspect, and drugs used for the treatment of mental illness may interfere with sexual functioning
- The mentally ill are the target of concerns from the public and professionals about inappropriate sexual displays, which can range from clumsy and naive sexual exploration to potentially assaultative behaviour

Assessment

Like all psychiatric problems, the assessment of psychosexual difficulties should be approached from biological, psychological and social perspectives. Sexual arousal arises from several components that are truly psychosomatic in terms of their interaction. Arousal usually involves a cognitive component involving a desire to have sexual relations, sexual fantasy or visualization, tactile sensations from skin, other influences such as the smell of perfumes, and physiological responses indicating arousal and enabling sexual intercourse; these can interact in any order and some may be more important than others to specific individuals. Assessment should be directed to all of these.

Physical illnesses frequently have an adverse effect on sexual functioning, and these should be excluded through a detailed history and physical examination. The history and physical examination should attend especially to the detection of arterial disease, diabetes and sensory neuropathies.

Examination of the genitals should be carried out early by an experienced clinician, preferably of the same sex as the patient, to exclude local pathology such as genital warts, phimosis, vaginismus and testicular pathology. A detailed drug history should be obtained (covering prescribed and illicit drugs and including alcohol), along with an assessment of personality and relationship history. The timing of onset is of particular importance, as disorders of sudden onset at the time of a stressor are generally considered to be psychological in origin. Disorders of more insidious onset may point to potential organic causes, especially if there are abnormal findings on physical examination.

The management of most psychosexual disorders includes intervening in the psychosomatic cycle of performance anxiety and poor performance. A Masters and Johnson approach is most commonly advocated and includes a behavioural approach with clear homework tasks based on mutually agreed goals. This involves an initial ban on sex to break the psychosomatic cycle. Graded exposure is a technique whereby each partner learns to rediscover what actually arouses them starting with just non-genital touch and massage. This needs to be carefully planned during homework sessions to ensure that there are no interruptions; both partners must make sure they are available and must see the session times as protected time into which no other business intrudes. Spending this time together on non-sexual matters also aids communication. Gradually focused genital sensation is reached by mutual agreement. The usual difficulty is to ensure that the pace is kept slow so that a couple do not miss out the non-genital components. Help with negotiation and communication further helps each of the partners to frankly discuss how they are feeling and which behaviours they wish were different.

Specific disorders

Erectile failure

This is defined as persistent failure to sustain an erection of sufficient rigidity for penetrative intercourse. The prevalence is associated with age and affects up to one-third of the over-65s. Erectile failure may have many causes, including psychological, neurological, vascular or endocrinological disorders, trauma, iatrogenesis and the use of alcohol and non-prescribed drugs. It has been estimated that up to 30% of men, and 50% of those aged 50–70, suffer from erectile dysfunction.

Peripheral nerve lesions (especially of sacral outflow S2–4), including cauda equina lesions and other types of CNS pathology (such as multiple sclerosis or spinal cord lesion) can cause erectile failure. Testosterone levels are rarely too low but there is an age-associated decline. Low testosterone usually affects the sex drive but is not solely responsible for erectile failure. High serum prolactin levels also affect libido, and can be the side-effects of prescribed medications (always consider this and consult the *British National Formulary*). Individuals with existing cardiovascular disease or risk factors for this (diabetes, hypertension, smoking, family history of heart disease and risk factors, high lipid levels) are especially likely to develop erectile failure of vascular origin. Psychogenic erectile failure usually arises suddenly, with normal ejaculation and continuing early morning erec tions. Erectile failure may also abate with another partner or during masturbation. Organic causes usually take effect slowly and, classically, early morning erections are absent.

Drugs associated with erectile failure include:

- Antihypertensives
- Antidepressants
- Antipsychotics
- Lithium
- Steroids
- Oestrogens
- Cimetidine.

Treatment should be directed at the cause of the erectile dysfunction and often requires effective liaison with the endocrine, medical, neurology and urology specialists. Blood chemistry, including glucose, urea and electrolytes and thyroid function should be investigated.

In some instances, intracavernosal injections of papaverine may be used as a diagnostic test, to exclude a vascular cause. This can be continued as a treatment but may produce fibrosis when administered chronically, and there is a risk of priapism. Patients need to be trained to self-administer safely and only those experienced in its use should offer it as a treatment, if all other interventions fail. Intracavernosal papaverine may also demonstrate impalpable Peyronie's disease, as might Doppler imaging. Urological assessment may involve ultrasonography, which can identify potentially repairable venous leaks.

The treatment of erectile dysfunction was revolutionized by the licensing of sildenafil (Viagra) in 1998, which was accompanied by protests at the attempts of the UK government to ration its prescription on the NHS. Sildenafil was the first simple-to-take oral treatment for erectile dysfunction and shortly after its release became the fastest-selling drug ever in the USA, with sales in excess of $1 billion in 1999 alone. At least three randomized trials have shown that sildenafil is clinically effective. In contrast to many other treatments, the erectile effects of sildenafil are dependent on sexual arousal, creating a more 'natural' erectile response. Despite reports of headache and flushing, sildenafil appears safe, with no evidence of serious cardiovascular side-effects. It does not cause priapism. There is some early evidence that sildenafil may increase sexual arousal in women. Despite the evidence of its effectiveness, sildenafil may only be prescribed on NHS prescriptions for those whose erectile dysfunction is due to prostatectomy, radical pelvic surgery, spinal cord injury, diabetes, multiple sclerosis or other serious neurological disease. This remains a matter of controversy, given the implication that this is a 'lifestyle' drug and therefore largely outside the remit of the National Health Service.

Other treatments for erectile dysfunction include urethral suppositories (alprostadil), vacuum devices and surgical implants. These treatments may be indicated in certain circumstances, such as young men with spinal cord injury or those unable to tolerate the side-effects of sildenafil.

Premature ejaculation

This is defined as ejaculation that seems involuntary and occurs before both partners are sexually satisfied. There is no magic time against which 'premature' is measured and this disorder may be better defined as a mismatch between partners during sexual activity. Performance anxiety after a single episode may compound and hence perpetuate the problem. Premature ejaculation is of course common among the young and sexually inexperienced and is not a sign of organic illness. It must be distinguished from retarded or absent ejaculation, which can arise in diabetes, neurological disorders (multiple sclerosis, spinal cord lesions, neuropathies), after prostatectomy and as a result of prescribed medication. Again, neuroleptic drugs, especially thioridazine, may be implicated.

Anorgasmia

This is defined as persistent failure of orgasm despite normal arousal. The time required for women to become sufficiently aroused varies and is usually longer than in men. Partner arousal time mismatch may be responsible. Some require manual clitoral stimulation before intercourse. The ability to reach an orgasm manually or with other partners makes it more likely that there is an arousal time mismatch rather than orgasmic failure. Anorgasmia is especially common in young women. An assessment includes physical examination for chronic gynaecological disorders such as vaginitis, endometriosis and pelvic inflammatory disease and also for the following:

- General physical illness
- Endocrine: adrenal insufficiency, diabetes, pituitary failure, hypothyroidism
- Drugs: antipsychotics and antidepressants (especially SSRIs)
- Spinal cord lesions and other serious neurological disorders

Anorgasmia in men needs to be distinguished from retrograde ejaculation and absent ejaculation. It is uncommon and is often associated with prostatic surgery or pelvic injury.

Vaginismus

This is defined as painful spasm of the pelvic floor muscles that prevents penetration. It should be distinguished from vaginal or pelvic infection, and from failure of vaginal lubrication. Usually vaginismus arises in young women with no sexual experience at their first attempt at intercourse; even passing the tip of the finger into the vagina results in spasm. This is often repeated at the time of vaginal examination. After excluding organic and psychological causes (including relationship difficulties) that may need attention in their own right, treatment involves increasing grades of dilator from small to large to expose the woman gradually to penetration. The longer the dilator is retained the further the spasm diminishes.

SLEEP PROBLEMS

Insomnia

Although individual requirements for sleep are highly variable, one-third of adults report problems falling asleep. Almost 40% of the elderly have disrupted sleep patterns. Insomnia can be mild and related to shift-work or acute stress; serious illness or persistent stress leads to longer-term sleep disturbance. Most psychiatric disorders, and many physical ones, are associated with disturbance of sleep. It is therefore important to take a careful history before embarking on any treatment. Those who are chronically poor sleepers may have severe anxiety and depressive disorders, chronic pain or severe physical illness.

Basic treatment involves improving sleep hygiene, and it is often helpful to outline the principles of this to patients who complain of difficulty sleeping. Individuals should be advised to avoid stimulants (including tea, coffee, alcohol and many soft drinks), especially in the evenings, and to keep to regular times for sleep and waking. It is important to remind individuals that they should get up if they find themselves in bed and unable to sleep, returning only when they feel tired. Under no circumstances should they compensate for a poor night's sleep by staying in bed, or napping, the next day. It is important to prepare for sleep by ensuring that the bedroom is comfortable, and that enough time is allowed to 'wind down' at the end of the day. A warm bath and a milky drink may help. Regular daytime exercise is also important. Many people worry about sleeping, and this makes it less likely that they will sleep.

Narcolepsy (hypersomnia)

Narcolepsy is defined as: (1) excessive daytime sleepiness (associated with napping); (2) cataplexy (a loss of muscle tone triggered by emotional arousal, causing immobility for up to minutes at a time); (3) hypnagogic hallucinations (vivid auditory or visual phenomena occurring at the onset of sleep); and (4) sleep paralysis (an inability to move on first waking). Occupational or social functioning are often compromised as a result of these difficulties.

Narcolepsy usually begins in adolescence and there is an equal male to female ratio. The prevalence is about 0.05%. Presentation is most common between the ages of 20 and 40 years. HLA typing reveals the DQB1 0602 subtype in 90% of sufferers. The primary pathology is thought to lie in the dysregulation of REM sleep, which is normally associated with dreaming and motor inhibition to prevent the dreams from being acted out. In narcolepsy there is a rapid transition from wakefulness to REM sleep. Differential diagnosis includes mental illness (depression, or schizophrenia if hallucinating), epilepsy (including temporal lobe or complex partial seizures), sleep apnoea and organic factors (e.g. hypothyroidism). Investigations in sleep laboratories may establish the REM latency, and video recordings help with the differential diagnosis of other sleep disorders (such as nightmares and sleepwalking). Investigation of possible narcolepsy includes polysomnography (monitoring of cardiovascular, respiratory and electrophysiological functioning during sleep) and the multiple sleep latency test (carried out after polysomnography and involving the quantification of daytime sleeping).

Tricyclic antidepressants and SSRIs reduce the frequency of attacks of cataplexy, and stimulants including dexamfetamine, methylphenidate and modafinil reduce the frequency and intensity of sleep attacks.

Nightmares

These are characterized by emotional and physiological arousal but with the loss of muscular tone (paralysis) characteristic of REM sleep. The subject will remember being unable to move as he/she wakes. The dream is vivid and remembered on wakening. The dreamer may be a little confused on wakening.

Night terrors

These occur in slow-wave sleep (usually stage 4) and hence start within a couple of hours of sleep onset. They are unusual in adulthood but can occur at times of stress. Children usually grow out of them.

Partial arousal from sleep is accompanied by intense fear, associated with psychological responses to fear: tachycardia, hyperventilation, perspiration. They can be precipitated by external noise or internal states. These same states may repeatedly trigger the episodes in one individual. Head injury, systemic illness (especially febrile states), drug and alcohol intoxication may be of importance in their onset in some individuals. There may be a series of screams or groans and physical movement may be that of escape activity, although usually the person simply sits in bed. Occasionally, violent acts can be carried out, but this is unusual.

Sleepwalking

Sleepwalking usually starts in childhood and adults subject to it usually sleepwalk, as in the case of night terrors, at times of stress, during drug and alcohol intoxication and after head injury. It usually occurs within the first few hours of sleep onset. There may be small repetitive movements of the sleepwalker, who can wander around the bedroom or even outside by negotiating barriers like doors, etc. There is then invariably a danger that the sleepwalker may injure themselves, walk into traffic, climb out of a window, etc. Contrary to popular opinion, sleepwalkers can carry out purposeful and complex acts that are responsive to their environment and only after careful observation may a patient's partner conclude that they are in fact asleep. There is often a family history. Management involves avoiding stressors, knowing triggers for that individual (alcohol for example), sleep hygiene and avoiding medication if possible. Benzodiazepines may exacerbate sleep apnoea and can produce hangover effects, dependency and rebound anxiety.

LEARNING DIFFICULTIES

DEFINITION

There has been considerable debate in recent years over the most appropriate nomenclature for this group of disorders, which have been referred to in the past as imbecility, feeble-mindedness, mental subnormality, mental deficiency, mental retardation and mental handicap, as well as learning disability and learning difficulties. Although 'learning difficulties' is generally preferred by health professionals, users and carers in the UK, ICD-10 (F70–79) classifies these conditions under the general heading of 'mental retardation'.

According to ICD-10, mental retardation is defined as a condition of *incomplete* mental development, as distinct from a *deterioration* in psychological or social functioning (as in dementia). The cardinal feature of mental retardation is 'a reduced level of intellectual functioning resulting in a diminished ability to adapt to the daily demands of the normal social environment'. Mental retardation is therefore characterized by deficits in motor, cognitive, linguistic and social skills compared with population norms. The clinical features of these disorders must be present before adulthood.

ICD-10 subdivides the continuum of impaired intellectual functioning into four categories of mental retardation: mild (F70), moderate (F71), severe (F72) and profound (F73).

Table 7 Prevalence of learning difficulties

Level	IQ	Proportion of population (%)	Proportion of those with mental retardation (%)
Mild	50–69	1.5	80
Moderate	35–49	0.3	12
Severe	20–34	0.2	7
Profound	<20	0.05	1

CLINICAL FEATURES

A definite diagnosis of mental retardation requires evidence of a reduced level of intellectual functioning compared with the appropriate population norm. Although it is tempting to make this judgement solely on the basis of IQ score, it must be remembered that intelligence is not a unitary construct. Thus, there may be significant discrepancies between skill levels in different domains of functioning. The assessment of intellectual functioning should be based on as many sources of information as possible, and should involve formal psychometric testing, including standardized, individually administered IQ tests. According to ICD-10, only a provisional diagnosis is permissible in the absence of standardized assessment procedures.

Mild mental retardation (F70) (IQ 50–69)

Characterized by delay in skill acquisition. Most mildly retarded individuals are able to function at a sufficient level to achieve full independence as adults, including eating and self-care (washing, dressing and toileting). Although conversational language is usually satisfactory, academic school work is usually significantly below average, with particular deficits in reading and writing. Individuals with mild mental retardation are often capable of maintaining semi-skilled employment that requires practical abilities but not written language skills. Social and emotional handicaps may or may not be overtly noticeable.

Moderate mental retardation (F71) (IQ 35–49)

Marked delay in the acquisition of language skills, with limited eventual achievement in this area. Achievement of other skills, notably self-care, is also impaired. Acquisition of language skills is variable. While academic school work is significantly below normal, many may acquire basic literacy skills. As adults, moderately mentally retarded individuals are able to do simple practical tasks, although these usually need to be highly structured. Complete independent living is rarely achieved. Although fully mobile, interpersonal social skills may be grossly limited. Discrepant profiles of abilities are common.

Severe mental retardation (F72) (IQ 20–34)

Similar clinical picture to that observed in moderate mental retardation, although with generally lower levels of social and intellectual functioning. Most people in this category also suffer from impaired motor function, indicating significant damage or abnormal development of the CNS (e.g. spasticity and athetosis).

Profound mental retardation (F73) (IQ less than 20)

Affected individuals are severely limited in their ability to comprehend and use language. Most are also immobile, incontinent and capable of little more than rudimentary non-verbal communication. Profoundly mentally retarded individuals are rarely able to perform any of the tasks involved in self-care, and therefore require continuous supervision.

EPIDEMIOLOGY

Although IQ test scoring is based on the assumption that intelligence is normally distributed, there are more people in the UK with an IQ below 70 than would be predicted on the basis of the normal distribution. The slight degree of skewing at the lower end of the IQ distribution is probably caused by the occurrence of pathological causes of low IQ (i.e. genetic causes) superimposed on a normally distributed characteristic in the general population.

Learning difficulties are more common in males, probably as a result of genetic abnormalities associated with the X chromosome. The prevalence of other psychiatric disorders (including the psychoses) is three to four times greater among individuals with learning difficulties than in the general population.

Epilepsy, and physical and neurological disabilities are very common in those with moderate, severe and profound mental retardation and the size of the association may well be directly related to the severity of intellectual impairment.

BASIC SCIENCES

In mild mental retardation there are usually no specific causes; these people represent the lower range of IQ distribution within the population. Where there is more than just a mild deficit, there is often an organic cause. The most common of these are:

- **Chromosomal abnormalities**: e.g. X-linked syndromes such as fragile X syndrome, Turner's syndrome, Klinefelter's syndrome and Down's syndrome, which affects 1:1000 live births
- **Genetic abnormalities**: e.g. phenylketonuria, homocystinuria, Tay–Sachs disease, Lesch–Nyhan disease, tuberous sclerosis, Niemann–Pick disease, Hurler's disease and neurofibromatosis
- **Intrauterine infection**: cytomegalovirus, rubella, syphilis, toxoplasmosis
- **Intrauterine insult**: fetal alcohol syndrome, heavy metal poisoning or teratogenic drugs
- **Endocrine disorders**: hypothyroidism
- **Neonatal trauma**: hypoxia or intraventricular haemorrhage from various causes, more common in premature delivery (cerebral palsy)
- **Cranial malformations**: hydrocephalus
- **Childhood infection**: meningitis, encephalitis
- **Childhood head injury**.

It is known from Rutter's work in the Isle of Wight that children who are of normal intelligence and brain-damaged are more likely to have psychiatric disorders. Epilepsy is especially linked to developmental abnormalities and low IQ. Furthermore, repeated seizures have been hypothesized to further damage neuronal tissue, although damaged tissue is also often the focus of seizures.

DIFFERENTIAL DIAGNOSIS

Those with learning difficulties can develop all the range of mental illnesses described elsewhere. Hence, one should consider the main groups of disorders. However, the assessment is usually complex and requires a careful appraisal of the context in which disturbed behaviour is displayed, as superficially similar behaviours might be attributable, after careful exploration, to hallucinosis or frustration in a depressed patient. A specialist team should be consulted. Assess physical impairments and sensory deficits. Many apparently unusual behaviours may be related to the difficult negotiation of development stages, perhaps to do with individuation, intimate sexual relationships and family relationships. Assessment is especially compromised when the IQ is less than 50 because of difficulties in communication.

MANAGEMENT

- The most important point to bear in mind is that there are three aspects of the problems experienced by patients: the impairment itself (e.g. organic brain damage), the disability (e.g. illiteracy) and the social handicap arising from the disability. While it is essential to try to identify the source of the impairment, by means of careful assessment, it is probably more important to consider the current needs of the patient and their carers. A careful developmental history should be undertaken, including all childhood investigations, with an outline of varying functional abilities and associated environmental and mental state findings. Family assessment is also essential

- **Psychological**: in the absence of effective communication, a behavioural analysis should be carried out, focusing on problem behaviours, their antecedents and consequences. It may be that it is only from the behaviour that one can ascertain the underlying mental state. Supportive counselling and frank discussion with a trusted professional are invaluable to aid assessment and enable the patient to get a better understanding and develop coping strategies. Family work is also important, especially after diagnosis or when the presentation changes and places the family in crisis also
- **Biological**: drug treatments are often used to control behaviour. These treatments are sometimes used without a good assessment of the underlying mental state. The response to medication is then (often erroneously) used to support a diagnosis. The safest antipsychotic to use is haloperidol. Benzodiazepines are also used acutely but for mood stabilization, irritability and manic states lithium and carbamazepine may be used to good effect. Lithium is also used to control unexplained states of self-mutilation and frustration leading to tantrums. Propranolol and clonidine also have been used to control self-destructive behaviours. Where there are specific symptoms of depression or where behaviour (e.g. crying, withdrawal) indicates depression, antidepressants should be prescribed
- **Social**: this involves the provision of support for families if the patient is still living with parents and/or siblings. More usually, it is necessary to ensure that an adequate level of supported housing is available. Those with major mental illness will need specialist supported housing where the staff are familiar with caring for the mentally ill as well as working and living with those with learning difficulties. Places of work and leisure are also necessary as part of an overall rehabilitation package

CHILD AND ADOLESCENT MENTAL HEALTH

OVERVIEW

A child presenting with difficulties should always be assessed within a developmental context, as part of a wider system of family, culture, educational establishment and social network.

The main patterns in presentation include disturbance in conduct (behaviour), emotions, relationships or development. The disturbance usually becomes apparent to others, typically parents, teachers, social workers or the police in the case of young offenders. They will then seek professional help. The problem therefore needs to be viewed as a disturbance not solely in the child.

In assessment, both the symptoms and the incapacity or impact of the symptoms must be considered. The safety of the child is paramount. Although confidentiality in the assessment procedure is important, information that puts a child at risk must result in the initiation of steps to ensure safety and protection.

A developmental and family history together with supplementary information from any relevant sources (e.g. school) is important. The assessment must ascertain whether the problem is apparent only in one situation or whether it is generalized. This will usually involve interviews with the family and child, and possible discussions with others who know the child. Further assessment (e.g. psychometric testing) may be required. Observation of behaviour is also helpful. The multiaxial diagnosis (ICD-10) takes account of the wider context and is a useful guide to the essential features of assessment.

- **AXIS I Clinical psychiatric syndromes**
- **AXIS II Specific disorders of development**
- **AXIS III Intellectual level**
- **AXIS IV Medical conditions**
- **AXIS V Associated abnormal psychosocial situations**
- **AXIS VI Global assessment of psychosocial disability**

EMERGENCIES

The acutely disturbed child or adolescent

A child or adolescent may present in a crisis, usually in a disturbed and agitated state. There may be a risk of violence, and the safety of the child and others will be of concern. It is important to establish a picture of the disturbance in the context of background history and any precipitating events. Organic aetiology, e.g. epileptic phenomena, diabetes, intoxication with drugs or alcohol, must be excluded. On rare occasions the disturbance may be due to an acute psychotic illness.

The first priority is safety. This requires that the child is placed in a setting that can contain the situation and where further observation, exploration and investigation is possible. Short-term use of sedation and anxiolytic treatment may be appropriate. A child and adolescent psychiatrist should be involved in the management.

Deliberate self-harm

Deliberate self-harm and suicide attempts are not infrequent in adolescence, particularly among girls. They usually present to A & E departments or GPs. It is important to be aware of particular risk factors. These include poverty, social deprivation, bullying, rural isolation and physical and sexual abuse.

Drug overdose is the most common method of self-harm, followed by cutting. Some young people may present having made threats only. Repeated cutting can be associated with a history of abuse and may be part of a picture of eating disorders, alcohol or substance abuse and other risk-taking behaviour. Drug overdoses are often related to relationship problems. There may be a serious lack of awareness of the potential dangers of over-the-counter medications such as paracetamol. Ideally, all young people who deliberately harm themselves should have a mental health assessment, and interventions to address the underlying problem should be offered. This is important, as there is an increased risk of further attempts and of completed suicide. The factors that are most likely to be associated with a higher risk of later suicide include:

- Male gender
- Older age
- High suicidal intent
- Psychosis
- Depression
- Hopelessness
- Having an unclear reason for the act of deliberate self harm.

The Mental Health Act 1983 and the Children Act 1989

The Mental Health Act 1983 and the Children Act 1989 will at times influence the management of children and adolescents with mental health problems. The relationship between the two is unclear and professionals often cannot decide which legislative scheme is appropriate for a particular child. Application of either Act requires careful consideration by both health services and social services.

The Children Act 1989 advocates a 'working together' approach that recognizes children's specific needs. The courts are often involved in decision-making. The Mental Health Act 1983 is often used in emergencies and when the diagnosis of a treatable mental disorder is clear.

The new Mental Health Act could be an opportunity to set out a new statutory scheme for the management of children and adolescents with mental health problems.

LIAISON BETWEEN CHILD AND ADOLESCENT PSYCHIATRY AND OTHER SERVICES

Acutely disturbed children and adolescents may present at A & E departments. In the initial assessment it is important to establish a precipitating factor for the disturbance and to exclude physical illness or organic causes. Often, an explanation for the disturbance can be identified and appropriate action can be taken to address the precipitants. Sometimes, admission for observation may be necessary. Other presentations include social problems (e.g. breakdown of family relationships) leading to a request for the child to be removed. In these circumstances it will be necessary to involve social services from the outset.

Paediatric liaison

Children under the age of 16 may occasionally be admitted to paediatric wards, either as emergencies or routinely. The principles for managing emergencies are essentially the same as for adolescents admitted to adult psychiatric wards, and close liaison between paediatric staff and child psychiatric staff is vital. In many instances there will be considerable overlap between psychological and paediatric medical problems. Joint approaches in management are the most effective.

Liaison with paediatric departments is a relatively well-established practice. This is also often of a multidisciplinary nature, involving input from social services. Psychosocial factors have a great influence on the wellbeing of a child and must be considered when addressing the needs of sick children if they are to be managed successfully.

Liaison with adult mental health services

Adolescents (aged over 16 years) may on rare occasions require admission to adult psychiatric wards, particularly as adolescent inpatient units are scarce. A joint care plan between adult psychiatric and child psychiatric services should ensure safety, containment, observation, assessment and emergency treatment. Ideally, the young person should be transferred to an adolescent inpatient facility as soon as possible for ongoing treatment.

Another important area is the management of children whose parents have mental illness. Parental mental illness has an impact on the care of their children, and on their development, and increases the risk of them developing mental health problems.

Working in the community

Multidisciplinary teams from specialist (tier 2 and tier 3; Together We Stand HAS 1995) departments provide these services. They are often made up of staff employed by different agencies, namely health, education and social services. The teams provide assessment, treatment, liaison, consultation and training. The settings in which they work vary from the central department to schools, homes or other venues in the community. As well as direct work with children and families, the teams also work with professionals from many different agencies who may be involved with the children. These include social workers, teachers, community nurses, GPs, paediatricians, speech and other therapists, the police and staff from adult community mental health teams and from voluntary and charitable agencies.

COMMON MENTAL HEALTH PROBLEMS OF CHILDHOOD AND ADOLESCENCE

Emotional disorders

Depression

Epidemiological studies show that many children are miserable. In the Isle of Wight studies, about 10% of 10-year-olds were miserable according to their parents, and over 40% of 14-year-olds were miserable by their own account. Depression presents in different ways at different developmental stages: preschool children often experience despair if separated from their attachment figures. From about the age of 6 years, the phenomenology of depressive disorders begins to resemble that of adult depression, and similar diagnostic criteria are therefore applied. In childhood, depression may present as school refusal, friendship difficulties, irritability and somatic complaints. Suicidal thoughts can occur in quite young children but plans do not usually become potentially fatal until adolescence. The sex ratio for childhood depression is equal, with the adult female preponderance becoming evident in adolescence. Half of depressed children have at least one other psychiatric disorder, typically a conduct or anxiety disorder.

The role of medication in treatment is limited. Its use is more common in postpubertal children. Cognitive therapy is becoming more widely used, in addition to family and individual therapy and school liaison.

Mania

Classical mania is rare in childhood. Mania in adolescence initially may present as schizophrenia as first rank symptoms are often prominent. The presentation can change in subsequent illness episodes. Treatment usually involves a combination of medication, family and individual therapy. Rehabilitation is important in predicting prognosis and involves liaison with, social and voluntary agencies, education and primary care.

Anxiety disorders

Between 5 and 10% of children and adolescents may have clinically significant anxiety disorders. The three commonest are separation anxiety disorder (fear of separation, arising in early childhood, of an unusual severity, persisting to a developmentally inappropriate extent, associated with significant social dysfunction), simple phobias and generalized anxiety disorder. Anxiety disorders may present as school refusal, somatic disorders, poor self-confidence and poor school performance.

School attendance problems are relatively common in most childhood emotional disorders, and may also be caused by bullying and difficulties with scholastic achievement. The child may complain of headache or abdominal pain on school mornings. A mother may covertly encourage the child if she herself is reluctant to be separated from the child or has emotional or other problems. Treatment involves rapidly re-establishing a pattern of school attendance, including supportive therapy for the child and family, and dealing with any contributory problems at the school.

Conduct disorders

In ICD-10 these are defined as 'disorders characterized by a repetitive and persistent pattern of dissocial, aggressive, or defiant conduct'. The dissocial conduct may include lying, stealing, truancy, fire-setting, cruelty to animals and vandalism. The behaviour pattern needs to be enduring, i.e. of 6 months or longer, and should be more severe than expected for the developmental level of the child. Conduct disorders are associated with underlying brain damage, adverse social circumstances and a family pattern of harsh and inconsistent discipline with poor monitoring and little child-centred activity. Antisocial behaviour in children may be a developmental trait, starting with temper tantrums and possibly leading to criminality, alcoholism, unemployment and inability to form good quality relationships in later life.

Conduct disorder can be classified as:

- **Confined to the family context**
- **Unsocialized**: associated with significant pervasive abnormalities in the individual's relationships with other children
- **Socialized**: occurring in individuals who are generally well integrated into their peer group
- **Oppositional defiant**: usually in younger children, characterized by defiant, disobedient behaviour that does not usually include delinquent acts
- **Other/unspecified**.

Mixed conduct and emotional disorders are relatively common.

Treatment for conduct disorders involves family therapy, which may be based on modification of either the child's behaviours or parent–child interactions. It is often combined with social casework. Parenting programmes are also effective in addressing these disorders.

Relationship disorders

- **Sibling rivalry disorder** is an unusual degree or persistence of emotional disturbance following the birth of a younger sibling
- **Elective mutism** is an emotionally determined selectivity in speaking often associated with social anxiety, withdrawal, sensitivity or resistance
- **Reactive attachment disorder** involves persistent abnormalities in the child's pattern of social relationships, associated with emotional disturbance and reaction to changes in environmental circumstances. The syndrome often results from severe parental neglect or abuse
- **Disinhibited attachment disorder** consists of diffuse non-selective attachment behaviour, attention-seeking and indiscriminate friendly behaviour, sometimes with poorly modulated peer interactions, persisting beyond a developmentally appropriate age

Developmental disorders

Pervasive developmental disorders

These are characterized by qualitative abnormalities in reciprocal social interactions and in patterns of communication, and by a restricted, stereotyped, repetitive repertoire of interests and activities. These features are present in all situations.

- **Childhood autism**: autism is believed to be a genetically influenced neurodevelopmental disorder defined by abnormal or impaired development present before the age of 3 years and with characteristic abnormalities in communication, social interaction and restricted repetitive behaviours.

Atypical autism is marked either by a later onset or by abnormal functioning in only two of the three domains

- **Asperger's syndrome**: characterized by abnormalities in reciprocal social interaction with restricted or stereotyped interests, in the context of normal language and cognitive development. It may be associated with clumsiness and there is a strong association with depression in later life
- **Rett's syndrome**: this condition occurs in girls, with apparently normal early development followed by partial or complete loss of speech and skills in locomotion and hand use

Other childhood disintegrative disorders also show a period of apparently normal development followed by loss of skills in several areas of development.

Specific disorders of psychological development are coded on axis II and include articulation disorder, expressive and receptive language disorders, specific reading, spelling and arithmetic disorders (including dyslexia) and specific developmental disorder of motor function.

Management involves coordination of many agencies, including health, social services and education, to address behaviour, support children and family and promote development.

Other psychiatric disorders in children and adolescents

Psychoses

Schizophrenia may present in childhood but is more common in adolescence. The dearth of acute inpatient facilities for young adolescents is a nationwide problem. Initial presentation may be insidious, with gradual deterioration in functioning at school and in peer relationships, or very florid, where a differential diagnosis of substance misuse should be considered.

Hyperkinetic disorders

These are believed to be of neurodevelopmental aetiology and are characterized by early onset, lack of persistence in activities that require cognitive involvement, and a tendency to move from one activity to another without completing any one. Activity is often excessive and disorganized, and affected children may be accident-prone, reckless and likely to form socially disinhibited relationships with adults. Disciplinary problems are common, as are difficulties in motor and language development and scholastic skills. Hyperkinetic disorders are more common in boys and may be associated with aggression, mild mental handicap, epilepsy and minor motor abnormalities. Treatment usually involves behavioural modification, with special teaching methods.

Careful use of a cerebral stimulant, such as methylphenidate, may bring relief to the level of a child being able to concentrate at school. Side-effects include appetite suppression, stunted growth and addiction, and monitoring must therefore be ongoing and careful.

Substance misuse

This is relatively common in adolescence and includes glue-sniffing, tobacco and alcohol consumption and use of illicit substances such as marijuana, cocaine, crack and Ecstasy. Peer and cultural pressures play an important part in establishing a pattern of substance misuse. Educational programmes have been designed to raise awareness among teachers and parents of the symptoms and signs of intoxication, and to educate youngsters on the detrimental effects of such substances. Substance misuse is more common in children with a history of conduct disorder.

Eating disorders

Anorexia nervosa, in particular, often begins in adolescence, and is dealt with more fully on pages 168–174. Family therapy is usually the treatment of choice.

Obsessive–compulsive disorder

Obsessive–compulsive disorder may have an early onset, particularly with obsessive ruminations or obsessive neatness. Obsessional traits are common in younger children. Persistent symptoms of OCD can be complex. Treatment may involve a combination of family or individual therapy, behaviour modification and medication.

Adjustment disorders and post-traumatic stress disorder

These conditions may go undiagnosed. Death of a parent or divorce may also involve disruptions to caring, possibly a move of home or school, and can result in significant emotional disturbance.

Sleep disorders

Disorders of sleep are common in childhood and include sleepwalking; sleep terrors and nightmares. Sleepwalking usually occurs during the first third of sleep, involves low levels of awareness and reactivity, and there is no recall of the event upon waking. Sleep terrors are very worrying to parents, involving terror, vocalization and motility. They usually occur in the first third of sleep and recall on waking is very limited.

Trichotillomania

This is a disorder characterized by hair loss due to recurrent failure to resist the urge to pull out hairs. It occurs more commonly in girls and is associated with mounting tension succeeded by a sense of relief following the hair pulling. Treatment should target the underlying anxiety and usually involves cognitive behaviour therapy.

Tic disorders

These involve involuntary, rapid, recurrent, non-rhythmic motor movements or vocal production. Gilles de la Tourette's syndrome is the most severe manifestation, comprising multiple tics and compulsive utterances. Treatment with haloperidol and behavioural interventions may be effective.

Enuresis

Enuresis is involuntary voiding of urine that is abnormal in relation to the individual's mental age and not secondary to an organic problem. A behavioural regimen is often used in treatment, involving star charts and bell-and-pad mechanisms. Use of tricyclic antidepressants may be successful for short critical periods such as family holidays.

Encopresis

Encopresis is the voluntary or involuntary passage of faeces in inappropriate places. It can occur monosymptomatically or as part of a wider disorder of emotions or conduct. Treatment involves ruling out an organic cause, addressing underlying disturbance and behavioural management.

CHILD ABUSE AND NEGLECT

Child abuse is an increasingly recognized problem and may be physical, sexual or emotional in nature. Most child abuse is carried out by parents or close relatives or carers. Many perpetrators have a history of being abused themselves and they are often socially disadvantaged. Children who are handicapped in some way are more likely to be abused. Abuse of any form may present as withdrawal or fearfulness, as an emotional or conduct disorder or as poor functioning at school.

Physical abuse, 'non-accidental injury', may present as broken bones, retinal haemorrhage or cigarette burns. The child may be retarded in mental, physical or social development. Sexual abuse is likely to be concealed and children may be coerced into secrecy with threats. Most victims are girls and their assailants are usually known to them. Boys are abused more commonly by strangers or by persons in authority. The presentation is often indirect, such as by running away from home, emotional or schooling difficulties or genital infection. Cases of child sexual abuse may not present until adulthood through self-injurious behaviour, psychosexual difficulties or emotional or personality disorders. Emotional abuse includes neglectful parenting and being habitually critical and rejecting, and the child may present with developmental delay or disordered behaviour.

If a doctor suspects abuse s/he should disclose concerns to a statutory agency such as social services, the NSPCC or the police. The Area Child Protection Committee will have a policy on who has responsibility for convening conferences – preliminary consultation to test the professional hypothesis, strategy discussions and child protection conferences.

The Children's Act 1989 outlines the procedures to be followed in suspected abuse cases. The main principles are:

- The child's welfare is paramount
- Parents have responsibilities to their children and have to be kept informed about their children and participate in decision-making
- Wherever possible, children should be cared for within their own families
- Children should also be kept informed and participate in decision-making about their future
- As far as the courts are concerned, an order for care under the Act should only be made if it would be better for the child than making no order at all; any delay in proceedings is likely to prejudice the child's welfare; in disputed cases the court must have regard for the child's wishes and feelings.

Child sexual abuse

Definition

> The involvement of dependent, developmentally immature children and adolescents in sexual activities they do not truly comprehend, to which they are unable to give informed consent; or which violate social taboos or family roles.

The acts of abuse can involve exposing children to watching sexual acts or involving them in one. Reports to date include oral, anal and genital intercourse and rape. Ritualistic and sadistic practices have been described.

Epidemiology

The incidence and prevalence data are not reliable, although some studies indicate that 10% of the adult population admit to sexually abusive experiences as children. The younger the child the less likely it is that they can verbalize their experience and the more likely that a change in behaviour will be the main indications. If family members are involved or threats have been made, feelings of shame, guilt and a fear of damaging others may delay disclosure.

Disclosure triggers

- Child's report
- Changes in behaviour
- Physical symptoms (vaginal sores, discharge, bleeding, anal bleeding and perineal tears) and injuries
- Sexually precocious behaviour and play inconsistent with the child's age; sexual preoccupations
- Allegation by parent, family member, school teacher, doctor
- Change in performance at school
- Depression
- Severe anxiety symptoms
- Acting out, deliberate self-harm, suicidality
- Anorexia
- Drug and alcohol misuse
- Prostitution

Risk factors for child sexual abuse

- Parents or carers have had abusive experiences
- Previous abusive experience
- Other types of abuse (emotional, non-accidental injury)
- Parental discord including sexual and marital difficulties
- Alcohol or drug misuse by parent or carer
- Perpetrator has a history of paedophiliac or sexual offences

Assessment

Assessment should involve an experienced child health professional. When professionals have concerns about the possibility of child sexual abuse they should always alert social services. Joint assessments, led by social services, include an assessment of parenting and child-rearing skills, problem-solving within the family and discovering and communicating the wishes of the child. Hurried intervention should be avoided as it may in fact cause harm. It is rare for a child to be removed from parents in an emergency. This might happen if the child disclosed the perpetrator and a return home would expose the child to further abuse or maltreatment, or if there was severe emotional and physical damage.

PSYCHIATRIC DISORDERS IN LATER LIFE

OVERVIEW

The relative and absolute size of the elderly population, in the UK and worldwide, is steadily increasing. There are currently 12 million people in the UK aged 60 and over (20% of the population), and this figure is estimated to rise to 18.6 million (30% of the population) by 2031.

- **Life expectancy at birth in 1991 was 73.2 years for men and 78.7 years for women**
- **People aged 65 and over as a proportion of the general population in the UK: 16%**
- **People aged 85 and over as a proportion of the general population in the UK: 2%**
- **People aged 65 and over living alone: 34%**
- **People aged 65 and over restricted by handicap: 13%**
- **People aged 65 and over comprise approximately 30% of all psychiatric admissions and 30% of community care referrals**
- **People aged 65 and over living in residential/nursing facilities: 4%**
- **Psychiatric disorders in later life can occur as de novo conditions or can be the result of chronic, long-standing conditions acquired in earlier years**
- **Prevalence of the more common psychiatric disorders in people aged 65 and over:**
  - Dementia: 5%, rising to 25% among those over 85
  - Depression: 9.8–22%
  - Anxiety disorders: 1.4–4.6%
  - Alcohol misuse: 5–12% of men and 1–2% of women
  - Late-onset schizophrenia: 0.3%

Psychiatric services for older people

Special psychiatric services for the elderly were first developed in the UK in the 1970s. These early services targeted older people with chronic mental illness starting in early life who had been treated in large institutions, those with functional mental illness and those with organic brain disease (mainly dementias).

Mental health services for older people should aim to:

- Promote and help regain or maintain independence and optimal functioning in the older person's home for as long as possible
- Respond promptly to medical and social problems, and liaise closely with primary care and other medical services for older people
- Provide multidisciplinary team input to address patients' physical, psychological and social needs
- Liaise with statutory, voluntary or private facilities/organizations to optimize the range of services available to an individual
- Provide treatment in a range of settings, including independent and supported accommodation and day care
- Support relatives caring for older persons at home.

The Royal College of Psychiatrists' recommendations for care (1992) suggested the following for a population of 10 000 people aged 65 and over:

- 10 acute beds with high staff–patient ratio
- 25–30 long-stay beds, including respite care
- One consultant old age psychiatrist
- One multidisciplinary team, including medical and nursing staff, occupational therapist and social worker

Psychiatric assessment in older people

In this age group a first assessment of the patient in their own home is preferred and should include:

- Recent psychiatric history (as in younger patients)
- Collateral history from a relative or carer is important, and essential in the presence of cognitive impairment
- Past psychiatric and medical history, including current medications and odd or uncharacteristic behaviours
- Assessment of current functional abilities, especially daily living skills, mobility and capacity for self-care
- Mental state examination, paying particular attention to cognitive abilities, including higher cortical functions (Mini Mental State Examination), as well as affective disturbances, suicidality and psychotic phenomena. Odd behaviours or abnormal movements may be observed during the interview
- Social history, including details about the patient's social circumstances, financial state, accommodation and support network
- Hazards in the home, e.g. ability to handle gas, fire or electrical appliances safely
- Any behavioural disturbance outside the home, e.g. wandering
- Complete physical examination assessing all systems, with particular attention to neurological examination.

Physical treatments in older people

- Older people have an increased sensitivity to drugs resulting from age-related changes in pharmacodynamics and pharmacokinetics, including protein binding
- Lowest effective dosage of medications is required and titration should be less rapid than in younger patients
- Non-compliance may be present, particularly in socially isolated, sensorily impaired or confused patients
- Polypharmacy should be avoided, since drug interactions may occur and further impair functioning and mental state
- Changes in mental state and behaviour (sometimes acute confusional states) may result from drug toxicity, which needs prompt intervention
- Drugs that increase the risk of falls (e.g. hypnotics) should be avoided if possible
- Drug-induced morbidity in this age group remains significant, particularly with antihypertensives, diuretics, hypnotics, antipsychotics, antidepressants, anxiolytics and antiparkinsonian drugs
- SSRIs should probably be used as first-line treatment because of their more favourable side-effect profile
- Atypical antipsychotics (e.g. risperidone and olanzapine) should be used in preference to older agents because of their more favourable side-effect profile. The older antipsychotics frequently cause extrapyramidal symptoms, hypotension and anticholinergic effects. Susceptibility to these increases with age. If needed, low doses (one-half to one-third of the younger adult dosage) should be prescribed
- Thioridazine should no longer be used because of cardiovascular side-effects, especially increased QT interval
- Lithium and sodium valproate may be used as mood stabilizers in older patients, but at lower doses than are commonly prescribed for younger adults
- Benzodiazepines and drugs with marked anticholinergic effects can cause drowsiness and confusion, leading to falls, incontinence and hypothermia. These should be avoided

Psychotherapy

- This is less widely available than in younger age groups and less well supported by evidence of effectiveness. Supportive, family, cognitive and behavioural approaches as well as more specific reality orientation therapy have been found to be helpful
- Psychodynamic psychotherapy is a more recent addition to psychological treatments in older people

Social support

- Basic measures should aim at reducing dependency, e.g. promoting self-care and domestic skills, encouraging social contact. Day centres, occupational

therapy and support at home may all be of some value, as may home improvements and aids
- Relatives may benefit from education and advice regarding the patient's condition and how best to manage it at home
- Practical help, including respite admission, day care and comprehensive home help are all valuable and enable many to remain at home with their families for longer

ABUSE AND NEGLECT OF OLDER PEOPLE

It is important to be aware of the possibility of abuse and neglect when planning care for someone suffering from dementia. Although often overlooked, abuse is estimated to affect at least 10% of those aged 65 and over. Variations include physical, psychological, financial and, rarely, sexual abuse. Violation of rights, neglect and acts of omission (e.g. withholding of food or medicine) also occur. Victims tend to be female, very old and frail, and more often suffer from physical or psychiatric illness. Perpetrators are usually related and financially dependent on the victim. Both victim and perpetrator tend to minimize the extent of the abuse. Caring for a demented person may predispose to abuse. Carer support and adequate management of the demented person are important in preventing abuse. Legal and housing issues may need to be considered in more severe cases.

COMMON PSYCHIATRIC DISORDERS IN OLDER PEOPLE

Dementia

Clinical features

Global deterioration of higher cortical function, manifesting as decline in memory, thinking, orientation, comprehension, language, intellect, personality and behaviour resulting from diffuse organic disease of the cerebral hemispheres or subcortical structures. Usually, but not necessarily, progressive and irreversible. Cognitive decline begins most commonly with deterioration in short-term memory and immediate recall, and progresses to global intellectual deterioration.

According to ICD-10, the primary requirement for a diagnosis of dementia is 'evidence of a decline in both memory and thinking which is sufficient to impair personal activities of daily living'. The symptoms of dementia must have been present for at least 6 months for a diagnosis to be made.

EARLY SIGNS AND SYMPTOMS

- Memory impairment for recent events and poor retention of new information: registers information but 5-minute recall impaired, although memory for distant events often preserved
- Reduction in range of interests
- Poverty of thought, perseveration and persecutory beliefs
- Subtle change in personality: may become irritable or aggressive, with occasional outbursts

- Changes in mood: anxiety and depression, or mood may be labile
- Change in behaviour: restless, distractible, sometimes antisocial (e.g. 'social lapses' such as shoplifting), rigid and stereotyped routines. May be suspicious and possibly physically aggressive and/or violent

Remember that the clinical features of dementia are influenced by premorbid cognitive/intellectual abilities and personality. Those with high premorbid IQ and/or good social skills may be able to compensate for early symptoms.

LATE SIGNS AND SYMPTOMS

- Further memory loss, including memory for distant events
- Disorientation, especially in time but also in place and, later, person; may lead to wandering
- Self-neglect and deterioration in self-care
- Restlessness, especially in the afternoons and evenings
- Dyspraxias, dysphasias and agnosias
- Mannerisms and stereotypies, including ceaseless pacing
- Incoherence or mutism
- Incontinence of urine and faeces

Epidemiology

Dementia is the most common psychiatric disorder among the elderly. The estimated prevalence of severe dementia is 3–5% among those aged over 65 and 20% among those aged 80 and over. The estimated annual incidence of severe dementia is 0.5–1.0% among those aged 70–79 and 2.0–2.5% among those aged over 80.

No consistent sex difference has been identified in the prevalence or incidence of severe dementia.

Mild dementia affects up to 10% of those over 65 years and 25% of those over the age of 80.

Basic sciences

Approximately 50% of all dementias are of the Alzheimer's type (ICD-10 F00), characterized by cerebral atrophy and enlarged ventricles on CT scan. Pathognomonic histopathological findings are a reduction in the number of neurones, accompanied by senile plaques (with beta-amyloid core), and neurofibrillary tangles (made of paired helical filaments). Cholinergic neurones are particularly affected, with evidence of reduced levels of acetylcholine and choline acetyltransferase. Cerebral changes are most prominent in the hippocampus, locus caeruleus and tempoparietal and frontal cortex.

The other main type of dementia identified is vascular dementia (ICD-10 F01), which includes multi-infarct dementia. In contrast to Alzheimer's disease, which has an insidious onset and progresses steadily over 2–3 years, vascular dementia tends to occur in the context of a history of transient ischaemic attacks or cerebrovascular accidents, and has a more 'stepwise' course.

For Alzheimer's disease, the main risk factors are a positive family history and advancing age. Recent research has identified an association between the presence of the gene responsible for apolipoprotein E (*ApoE*) and an increased risk of Alzheimer's disease. Although this association has been found in sporadic (non-familial) cases of Alzheimer's disease, it may be that the *ApoE* gene further increases the risk of Alzheimer's disease among those with a positive family history.

Dementia also occurs commonly among those with a history of severe and/or repeated head injury, such as boxers (dementia pugilistica).

Differential diagnosis of dementia

ORGANIC

- Normal ageing, which may mimic mild dementia, especially if the person is stressed
- Delirium (acute confusional state; see pp. 31–34). Likely to be associated with infection, e.g. respiratory tract infection. Diagnosis of acute confusional state supported by evidence of impaired level of consciousness, with lucid intervals and/or diurnal changes in symptom intensity. Delusions and/or hallucinations are common and are usually rich in ideas and associations and devoid of the negative affective flavour found in depression. Unlike dementia, symptoms are almost always reversible
- Amnesic syndrome (Korsakoff's syndrome) resulting from alcohol abuse and characterized by severe deficit in short-term memory and confabulation
- Reversible forms of dementia, including:
  - Multi-infarct dementia, associated with hypertension and characterized by focal neurological deficits, stepwise progression and pseudobulbar signs
  - Normal-pressure hydrocephalus, characterized by gait ataxia, incontinence and progressive dementia. May result from trauma, haemorrhage or infection. CSF pressure is normal but ventricles are dilated on CT scan
  - Drug intoxication, commonly iatrogenic: probable candidates are digoxin, benzodiazepines, analgesics and methyldopa
  - Subdural haematoma
  - Neoplastic space-occupying lesions
  - Metabolic disorders, particularly hypothyroidism
  - Vitamin B_{12} or folate deficiency
  - Hepatic or renal failure
  - Infectious causes – tuberculosis, toxoplasmosis, cerebral abscess or neurosyphilis

PSYCHIATRIC

Depression must *always* be considered, particularly where there is a history of 'acute' cognitive impairment. Cognitive impairment may be marked, because of severe psychomotor retardation, hence the name 'pseudodementia'. Unlike those with dementia, who may try to deny cognitive decline, elderly patients with depression complain of memory loss and difficulty with concentration

Management – biological

Once the clinical diagnosis has been made, it is essential to exclude potentially reversible causes of dementia. Basic investigations include full blood count, erythrocyte sedimentation rate (ESR), urea and electrolytes, liver function tests, thyroid function tests, vitamin B_{12} and folate, chest X-ray and ECG. CT scan or MRI is helpful to exclude space-occupying lesion and subdural haematoma.

For mild to moderate dementia of the Alzheimer's type (but with Mini Mental State Examination score above 12), consider treatment with acetylcholinesterase inhibitors, i.e. donepezil, rivastigmine and galantamine. These drugs improve cholinesterase transmission and delay the progression of the disorder. Typical average improvements of 1–2 points in MMSE score over 6 months are usual compared with placebo, although these effects are invariably temporary. Side-effects include nausea, vomiting, diarrhoea and abdominal pain. These drugs, although expensive, have been recommended by the National Institute for Clinical Excellence, with specific guidelines:

- Assessment and diagnosis must be made in a specialist clinic
- Treatment may only be initiated by a specialist
- Review must take place within 4 months, and treatment should be discontinued where there has been no evidence of clinical benefit
- These drugs are not indicated for individuals with MMSE scores below 10

Other physical treatments should also be considered, including low-dose sedating neuroleptics (preferably atypical drugs such as risperidone) for insomnia, restlessness, agitation, paranoia and/or aggressive behaviour. If markedly depressed, consider treatment with an antidepressant. Beware overuse of drugs: remember cardiovascular side-effects and the possibility of falls.

Management – social

The main aim of effective care is to provide good, safe physical care in an environment that is familiar to the individual for as long as possible. It is important to provide support for family and carers as well as for the individual with dementia. Respite care may be greatly appreciated.

Management – psychological

The aim is to allow the individual with dementia to maintain their self-esteem, thus avoiding traumatic catastrophic reactions. Such measures include discussions of past and current events, visible means of orientation and highly structured daily activities.

Delirium

Definition

Delirium is an acute organic brain dysfunction, characterized by disturbance of consciousness and attention, perception, thinking, memory, psychomotor activity and emotion, that is transient and of fluctuating intensity. Unlike dementia (see above) delirium is almost always non-progressive and reversible.

Clinical features

- Impairment of consciousness and attention. Disorientation for time, place and sometimes for person. Inability to attend to one stimulus for a prolonged period
- Illusions, hallucinations and delusional beliefs. Usually transient, fragmented and poorly systematized. Hallucinations may be visual as well as auditory
- Restlessness, overactivity and agitation. May, however, show signs of hypoactivity and psychomotor retardation. Speech may be increased or decreased
- Impairment of registration: very poor short-term memory
- Emotional disturbance: depression, anxiety and fearfulness are common. Mood may appear quite labile. Perplexity and suspiciousness are also seen
- Disturbance of sleep–wake cycle: manifests as insomnia, reversal of diurnal cycle, daytime drowsiness and worsening of symptoms at night
- Other signs of cerebral dysfunction including dysphasia, apraxia and dysgraphia

The onset of delirium is usually rapid.

Epidemiology

Seen most often in the elderly (> 60 years) and among hospital patients. Reported to occur in 10% of medical patients, 20% of burns patients and 30% of intensive therapy unit patients. 'Chronic' delirium lasting for 6 months or more has been observed among patients with chronic liver disease, carcinoma and subacute bacterial endocarditis. A previous episode of delirium significantly increases the risk of future delirium.

Basic science

Delirium is almost always due to an underlying systemic organic disturbance. Common causes include:

- **Infections**: e.g. respiratory or urinary tract infections, cellulitis and septicaemia
- **Cardiovascular disturbance**: arrhythmias, blood loss or anaemia (e.g. post-operative)
- **Respiratory distress or hypoxia**
- **Metabolic disturbances**: hypoglycaemia, renal or liver failure, severe vitamin deficiency
- **Neoplasms.**

Differential diagnosis

- Dementia (see p. 202)
- Acute psychotic disorders, including schizophrenia and mania
- Acute intoxication: drugs, alcohol or poisons, including Wernicke's encephalopathy (see pp. 134–149)
- Acute withdrawal from drugs or alcohol

- Temporal lobe epilepsy and postictal states
- Dissociative states

Management

The most important aspect of management is the identification of the cause of delirium. Many of the causes of delirium are life-threatening medical emergencies. Since the delirious patient is behaviourally disturbed it is easy to misdiagnose a primary psychiatric disorder. It is therefore imperative to physically examine and investigate any patient who is disorientated for time and place.

Physical examination

Look for evidence of focal sepsis, trauma, cardiac, renal or hepatic failure. Investigations should include urgent full blood count, urea and electrolytes, glucose, ESR, chest X-ray and blood cultures if pyrexial. EEG and CT scan are indicated if neurological signs are elicited or if no cause is found and symptoms persist.

Medical care

Should concentrate on treating the underlying cause of the delirium. Small amounts of neuroleptic medication (e.g. chlorpromazine) may help behavioural disturbances, including agitation and restlessness, as well as emotional lability, hallucinations and frightening illusions. Skilled nursing care is imperative. The delirious patient requires one-to-one nursing in a quiet but well-lit room. Staff should expect that the symptoms of delirium are likely to be worse at night than during the day.

AFFECTIVE DISORDERS IN THE ELDERLY

Unipolar depression

Clinical features

These are similar to the presentation in younger adults, but agitation and/or retardation are more common in this age group. Apathy, self-neglect and social withdrawal are also common, leading in some instances to life-threatening dehydration. Hypochondriacal preoccupations tend to be more common in depression among the elderly and may become delusional. Psychotic symptoms tend to occur more often than among younger depressed patients, and most often take the form of delusions of poverty, physical illness, nihilism, guilt, persecution.

Depression in the elderly has been referred to as 'pseudodementia', characterized by frequent 'don't know' answers, but no actual major memory impairment.

Epidemiology

The point prevalence of depression in people aged 65 and over is approximately 10%, 2–3% of which is severe. The prevalence is higher in females, as among younger adults, although this gender difference tends to diminish with age. The incidence of suicide also increases with age and is commonly associated with clinical depression. Nevertheless, depression tends to be poorly detected in primary care.

Aetiology

The risk factors for depression tend to be the same as those found for younger adults, although genetic factors appear to be less important. Physical illness, disability and social isolation appear to be especially important risk factors for depression in the elderly, and bereavement and other losses are important triggers.

Iatrogenic causes are important in this age group and include antihypertensive and other drug treatments.

Differential diagnosis

In dementia, cognitive difficulties usually precede mood disturbance. Depressed individuals usually exhibit partial cognitive deficits due to poor concentration rather than the global impairment associated with dementia.

Organic disorders must be excluded, including hypothyoidism and anaemia secondary to vitamin B_{12} or folate deficiency. Other organic conditions to be excluded include metabolic disorders, head injury and space-occupying lesions.

Paranoid states (including schizophrenia and delusional disorder) may have an affective component, although this is usually less prominent than in depression.

Management

- This is similar to the management of depression in younger adults. It is, however, important to pay particular attention to the assessment of physical health in the elderly
- Antidepressant treatment is usually effective but caution is needed because of the increased occurrence of side-effects. In particular, many antidepressants have cardiovascular side-effects and may cause arrhythmias. Interactions with other drugs are also important, given that many older people are on other forms of medication. It is therefore recommended that antidepressants should be started at lower doses than in younger adults. Following recovery, treatment with antidepressant drugs at therapeutic dose should be continued for at least 6 months, and for at least 1–2 years in those with recurrent depression
- Hospital admission is indicated if there is evidence of agitation, suicide risk or severe self-neglect
- Electroconvulsive treatment is indicated in severely agitated, retarded, stuporose patients and those who have not responded to an adequate trial of medication. It may have a more rapid effect than drug treatment and avoids the potentially severe side-effects of drugs. Periods between treatments should be extended for those with marked confusion following ECT
- Psychotherapy may be used as an adjunct to the above treatments or on its own for less severe illness. Approaches are similar to those offered in

younger age groups, comprising supportive, cognitive, group and family therapy. Bereavement counselling should be considered where appropriate
- Social interventions, including occupational therapy, and enhanced social support in and outside the home may be useful. The full range of treatment settings – day hospital, day centre, community (independent or sheltered/residential accommodation) – should be considered
- Prognosis is good initially (85% of inpatients recover) but the relapse rate is high. Over 60% of patients relapse within 3 years and 30% die within 6 years. Good prognostic factors include onset before age 70, absence of organic brain disease or serious physical illness, short duration of episode and good compliance and response to treatment

Bipolar affective disorder (mania)

Clinical features

Similar to younger age groups, but may be more irritable ('miserable mania') with less flight of ideas. May have a clinical presentation similar to that in acute confusional state.

Epidemiology

Manic episodes account for just 5% of affective disorders in those aged 65 and over. Incidence does not increase with age, unlike unipolar depression. It is rare for mania to present for the first time in old age.

Management

As for younger patients, albeit with appropriate caution when using drug treatments. Lithium prophylaxis is also effective in this age group, although serum levels should be maintained at the lower end of the younger adult therapeutic range to avoid toxicity. Remember that renal clearance falls with age.

Anxiety disorders

Clinical features

Similar to those in younger age groups. Phobic signs and symptoms tend to be less severe than in younger patients but equally debilitating. Older anxious patients often have prominent hypochondriacal symptoms.

Epidemiology

The prevalence of phobias in the elderly is 5–10%. Generalized anxiety disorder affects approximately 2–5% of those over 65, while the prevalence of panic disorder is about 0.1%. Aetiological factors include genetic vulnerability, early parental loss, chronic physical disability, poor social networks and an acute physical or traumatic event.

Management

As for younger age groups, the mainstay of treatment is cognitive behaviour therapy.

Schizophrenia in later life

Clinical features

Schizophrenia is seen most commonly in older people who have had this illness since early adulthood (early-onset schizophrenia). Although rare, schizophrenia may begin after the age of 40 (late-onset schizophrenia) or occasionally after the age of 60 (very-late-onset schizophrenia). The nosological distinction between these three conditions remains contentious and there certainly appear to be more similarities than differences between their clinical features. Unlike DSM-III, neither DSM-IV nor ICD-10 distinguishes types of schizophrenia on the basis of age of onset.

In very-late-onset cases, formal thought disorder and affective blunting are rare, while visual, tactile and olfactory hallucinations are more common than in cases of earlier onset. Very-late-onset schizophrenia (which was sometimes referred to in the past as (late) paraphrenia, is also characterized by paranoia, delusions of persecution and passivity phenomena. Common complaints concern surveillance and/or interference from neighbours. Mood is usually congruent with psychotic phenomena and may appear depressed. Self-neglect, abuse of neighbours and complaints to police are commonplace. It is said that personality remains well preserved in most cases.

Epidemiology

It has been estimated that up to one-quarter of all cases of schizophrenia begin after the age of 40. The total community prevalence for schizophrenia among those aged over 65 has been estimated at between 0.1% and 0.5%.

The epidemiological evidence supports a cut-off at age 60 for cases of very late onset, but provides little support for a distinction between cases that begin in early adult life and those beginning in middle age. Very-late-onset schizophrenia is more common in women. Associations have been reported between very-late-onset cases and both sensory impairment and social isolation.

Basic science

No differences have been found in the cognitive deficits associated with early- and late-onset cases. Brain imaging findings are essentially similar regardless of age of onset. Family studies have reported stronger familial aggregation of schizophrenia (i.e. risk of schizophrenia in family members) in early- and late-onset cases than in cases of very late onset. Some studies have found an increased familial risk for affective disorders in probands with schizophrenia of later onset.

Management

Patients with very-late-onset schizophrenia may be difficult to engage because of their paranoid symptomatology, which results in poor compliance with medication. Hospital admission for assessment and treatment is usually necessary (often compulsorily).

Antipsychotic medication, whether using typical or atypical agents, often leads to a reduction in the florid symptomatology, allowing the patient to return to premorbid functioning. However, encapsulated delusional beliefs tend to persist despite continuing antipsychotic treatment. Community services should strive to address patients' physical, psychiatric, psychological and social needs.

The effectiveness of psychosocial and behavioural interventions in very-late-onset schizophrenia have yet to be evaluated.

SECTION IX

Therapeutics

DRUG TREATMENTS

In this section a basic outline of clinical pharmacology is presented with an introduction about drug absorption, metabolism and excretion. For a more detailed discussion of individual drugs, readers are referred to the latest edition of the *British National Formulary*.

PHARMACOKINETICS

Pharmacokinetics is defined as the study of the absorption, distribution, metabolism and excretion of drugs. This includes the time frame over which these processes take place and the effects of ageing, disease states (particularly renal and hepatic impairment) and concomitant drug therapy. An understanding of pharmacokinetic processes and how these are altered by physical illness and other drugs encourages rational prescribing.

Absorption

Bioavailability

Bioavailability is a measure of the relative amount of administered drug that reaches the systemic circulation.

- **FACTORS INFLUENCING BIOAVAILABILITY**
  - Drug characteristics (e.g. lipid solubility)
  - Formulation characteristics (e.g. liquid, enteric-coated, slow-release)
  - Interactions (e.g. food or other drugs in gut)
  - Patient characteristics (e.g. gut disease – malabsorption, gut motility)
  - Route of administration (orally administered drugs are subject to first-pass metabolism, parenteral drugs are not)

Routes of drug administration

- **ORAL**
  - Most commonly used route
  - Bioavailability altered by the factors outlined above
  - Drug is subject to first-pass metabolism
- **SUBLINGUAL**
  - Rapid absorption
- **RECTAL**
  - Easy to use (e.g. diazepam in status epilepticus)
  - Useful when nausea is a problem or patient is 'nil by mouth'
  - Not liked by some patients
- **INTRAMUSCULAR**
  - Avoids first-pass metabolism, therefore lower dose required
  - Onset of action usually more rapid than oral route (although not true for diazepam)

- Absorption influenced by local blood flow (e.g. faster from arm than thigh)
- Affected by physical properties of the drug (e.g. phenytoin precipitates in muscle)
- Prolonged absorption with sustained-release (depot) preparations
- Compliance ensured
- Complications include skin necrosis, abscess, sterile nodules, fibrosis, nerve damage, pain, inadvertent intravenous injection, elevated creatine phosphokinase

INTRAVENOUS

- Bioavailability 100%
- Instantaneous response
- Rate of administration flexible
- Drug cannot be recalled if toxicity develops
- Only water-soluble drugs or emulsions can be given
- Local irritant properties of drug important
- Risks of anaphylaxis, infection, tissue damage, end-organ damage if administration too rapid

Most antidepressants and antipsychotics are lipid-soluble, poorly ionized in the gut and absorbed by passive diffusion, whereas lithium (not lipid-soluble) is ionized and absorbed by an active carrier system. Drug interactions with concomitant medications can slow down absorption from the gut (anticholinergic activity; antacids/food in stomach) or speed it up (thyrotoxicosis, gastroenteritis). Diazepam is slowly and erratically absorbed by the intramuscular route and lorazepam is the preferred drug for rapid intramuscular sedation.

Distribution and protein binding

Volume of distribution

This is a theoretical concept that assumes that the body is a single compartment in which the drug is evenly distributed. The volume of distribution is therefore equal to the amount of drug in the body divided by the plasma drug concentration. For highly fat-soluble or protein-bound drugs, this figure is large.

In fact, drugs are rarely distributed evenly throughout the body. Highly protein-bound drugs are susceptible to changes in binding state leading to toxicity as only free drug is biologically active. In low-protein states oral doses need to be decreased. Protein-bound drug might be displaced (e.g. anticonvulsants, antidepressants and neuroleptics). Lithium is not protein-bound and has a volume of distribution just larger than total body water. Anything affecting fluid balance (diarrhoea, diuretics) will therefore influence plasma lithium concentrations.

Metabolism

- **Phase 1**: Modification (oxidation, reduction, hydrolysis)
- **Phase 2**: Conjugation (with glucuronic acid, glycine, glutamine, sulphate, acetate)

Metabolic derivatives may be more or less active than the parent compound, with different half-lives; for example, amitriptyline is converted to nortriptyline, imipramine is converted to desipramine.

First-pass metabolism in the liver or gut wall is especially important if the drug is lipid-bound. Thus only 30% of an oral dose of chlorpromazine is absorbed because the rest is metabolized in the liver on first pass. Hence, if a lipid-bound drug is given parenterally, the dose needs to be reduced accordingly.

Pharmacogenetics

Slow and fast metabolism of some drugs (e.g. phenelzine) is influenced by acetylator status, which is genetically determined. Rapid acetylation has autosomal dominant inheritance. Its prevalence varies across ethnic groups (from 18% in Egyptians to 100% in Canadian Inuit).

Several of the hepatic cytochrome enzymes involved in drug metabolism exhibit genetic polymorphism. The most important are:

- CYP1A2 (metabolizes, for example, clozapine and olanzapine)
- CYP2C (metabolizes, for example, diazepam and tertiary amine antidepressants)
- CYP2D6 (metabolizes many antidepressants and antipsychotics).

Poor metabolizers at CYP2D6 (up to 10% of the population) show high blood levels of psychotropic drugs and are therefore more likely to have adverse effects. The elderly have a slower rate of metabolism and are more sensitive to the effects of a drug because of changes at receptor level and failing homeostatic mechanisms (pharmacodynamic effect).

Excretion

Half-life

Half-life is defined as the time taken for the blood concentration to diminish by 50%. Most drugs are eliminated by 'first-order kinetics': the amount of drug eliminated is proportional to the amount of drug there is in the body. It takes about five half-lives to reach steady state. This must be remembered when depot antipsychotics are prescribed, as plasma levels will continue to rise for several months after a dosage increase. The frequency of daily administration also is dictated by half-life: drugs with a short half-life need to be given more frequently. Clinically effective dosage schedules can therefore be worked out.

Clearance

Clearance is the volume of biological fluid cleared of drug per unit time. Age and renal disease can affect clearance.

Renal and hepatic function

Most drugs are eliminated by the kidneys as inactive metabolites after they have been conjugated. Lithium is excreted without any metabolic changes. Over 60% of lithium in the filtrate is reabsorbed in the proximal convoluted tubule and competes with sodium. Sodium depletion can therefore lead to lithium toxicity, as can concomitant treatment with diuretics or non-steroidal anti-inflammatory drugs (NSAIDs).

Liver disease impairs the breakdown of drugs and prolongs the effects of active drug. Enzyme induction speeds up, and enzyme inhibition slows down drug metabolism. Barbiturates and carbamazepine are inducers of liver enzymes.

Some SSRIs are potent inhibitors of CYP1A2, 2C, 2D6 and 3A4. Note that individual patterns of inhibition vary: fluoxetine and paroxetine are the most, and citalopram the least potent inhibitors of liver enzymes.

Significant interactions with other drugs (e.g. theophylline, phenytoin, warfarin) can therefore be anticipated.

SPECIFIC PSYCHOTROPIC DRUGS

Antipsychotics

Typical antipsychotic drugs have been available since the 1950s. They are mainly used to treat schizophrenia, organic psychoses and mania. All are equally effective but potency and side-effects differ. Their antipsychotic activity is mainly due to dopamine blockade. Sites of dopamine blockade (and effects) include: striatum (extrapyramidal symptoms and motor effects); limbic forebrain and neocortex (antipsychotic activity); hypothalamus (raised prolactin levels); and brainstem (antiemetic action on chemoreceptor trigger zone). Other side-effects are mediated via affinity for other receptor pathways, or are idiosyncratic.

All cause extrapyramidal side-effects (EPSEs) and raise serum prolactin.

Adverse effects

MOTOR MANIFESTATIONS

Including acute dystonias (10%), pseudoparkinsonism (20%), akathisia

Table 8 Antipsychotics: equivalent dose and adverse effect (from reference 3)

Drug	Equivalent (mg)	Sedation	Extrapyramidal side-effects	Anti-cholinergic	Cardio-vascular
Chlorpromazine	100	+++	++	++	+++
Promazine	200	+++	+	++	++
Thioridazine	100	+++	+	+++	+++
Fluphenazine	2	+	+++	++	+
Perphenazine	10	+	+++	+	+
Trifluoperazine	5	+	+++	+/–	+
Flupentixol	3	+	++	++	+
Zuclopentixol	25	++	++	++	+
Haloperidol	3	+	+++	+	+
Droperidol	4	++	+++	+	+
Pimozide	2	+	+	+	+++
Loxapine	10	++	+++	+	++

(25%) and tardive dyskinesia (5% per year of antipsychotic exposure). Tardive dyskinesia may be irreversible in 50% of cases

- **NEUROLEPTIC MALIGNANT SYNDROME**
  Occurs in 0.5% of newly treated patients; 20% mortality. Symptoms include hyperthermia, muscular rigidity, labile blood pressure, fluctuating consciousness, abnormal liver function tests, raised white blood count, raised creatine phosphokinase
- **HYPOTHALAMIC EFFECTS**
  Hyperprolactinaemia, impotence, galactorrhoea, gynaecomastia, hypothermia, heat stroke
- **SEDATION**
  Ataractic state, depression
- **ANTICHOLINERGIC EFFECTS**
  Diplopia, dry mouth, urinary retention, constipation, cardiac conduction block or delay, arrhythmias, confusion
- **ANTIADRENERGIC EFFECTS**
  α_1-receptor blockade leads to hypotension and tachycardia, nasal stuffiness, delayed or inhibited ejaculation, rarely priapism
- **LOWER SEIZURE THRESHOLD**
  Leading to epileptic fits. Dose-related and more common with sedative drugs.
- **INCREASED APPETITE AND WEIGHT GAIN**
  Atypical drugs are worse in this respect than the older drugs
- **CARDIAC ARRHYTHMIAS (VIA QTC PROLONGATION)**
  Dose-related. Greatest risk with low potency phenothiazines. Can be fatal. For this reason, both thioridazine and droperidol are due to be withdrawn and should be used with caution
- **ALLERGIC REACTIONS**
  Cholestatic jaundice, urticaria, dermatitis, blood dyscrasias, light-sensitive rash
- **RARE**
  Pigmentary retinopathy (especially thioridazine), corneal and lens opacities, raised cholesterol, diabetes

Management of adverse effects

- Choose a drug with the best side-effect profile that the individual patient can tolerate, but also to capitalize on the drug effects (e.g. sedation may be desirable)
- **Neuroleptic malignant syndrome**: stop all drugs, seek medical assessment, transfer to intensive therapy unit if severely ill and dehydrated. Combined administration of the muscle relaxant dantrolene and dopamine

Table 9 Depot antipsychotic drugs

Drug	Oil base	Test dose	Equivalent dose (2 weekly)	Recommended dosage interval (weeks)	Maximum BNF dose	Dose in elderly
Flupentixol	Coconut	20 mg/ 1ml	40 mg	1–4	400 mg/ week	Quarter to half dose
Fluphenazine	Sesame	12.5 mg/ 0.5 ml	25 mg	2–5	200 mg/ month	'Reduced dose'
Haloperidol	Sesame	25 mg/ 0.5 ml	50 mg	2–4	300 mg/ month	12.5–25 mg monthly
Pipothiazine	Sesame	25 mg/ 0.5 ml	25 mg	4	200 mg/ month	5–10 mg monthly
Zuclopentixol	Coconut	100 mg/ 0.5 ml	200 mg	1–4	600 mg/ week	Quarter to half adult dose

Adverse effects as for oral preparations, as well as injection site reactions (nodules, granulomas, abscess or fibrosis) in 20% of patients. The latter may be minimized by:
- Using the smallest volume. Concentrates where possible. No more than 2 ml per site
- At the lowest frequency. Avoid weekly injections if possible
- Using good injection technique
- Rotating injection sites

agonist bromocriptine reduces mortality and speeds up recovery in some cases but these drugs themselves carry considerable adverse effects. Rechallenge with an antipsychotic should be undertaken with great caution

- Most other side-effects can be dealt with by switching to another antipsychotic with a different side-effect profile. Weight gain can be difficult to manage
- **Motor symptoms**: switch to an atypical drug. If still problematic or switch not possible:
  - *Acute dystonias*: procyclidine (5–10 mg), orally, i.m. or slow i.v.
  - *Pseudoparkinsonism*: anticholinergics such as procyclidine or benzhexol
  - *Akathisia*: reduce neuroleptic dose; consider propranolol (20–40 mg twice or three times daily) or cyproheptadine (4–8 mg twice daily)
  - *Tardive dyskinesia*: stop anticholinergics, switch to an atypical antipsychotic (ideally clozapine), tertrabenazine may offer some relief

Atypical antipsychotics

Atypical antipsychotics cause fewer extrapyramidal side-effects than the older drugs but are not devoid of other side-effects. They all cause weight gain, which may be greater than with the older drugs, and some cause hyperprolactinaemia. Clozapine is the only antipsychotic proven to be effective in treatment-refractory schizophrenia. There is no evidence base to support the use of other atypicals in these patients.

While atypicals cause less secondary negative symptoms than the older drugs, there is no evidence to support superior efficacy in primary enduring negative symptoms.

Table 10 Atypical antipsychotics

Drug	Optimal dose	Maximum dose	Sedation	Anti-cholinergic	Postural hypotension	Prolactin elevation
Risperidone	4–6 mg	16 mg	+/–	–	++	Yes
Olanzapine	10–20 mg	20 mg	++	+	+/–	No
Quetiapine	300–450 mg	750 mg	+	+	++	No
Zotepine	Not determined	300 mg	++	++	++	Yes
Amisulpride	400–800 mg	1200 mg	+/–	–	–	Yes
Sulpiride	Not determined	2400 mg	+/–	–	–	Yes
Clozapine	Average 450 mg	900 mg	+++	+++	+++	No

Risperidone commonly causes EPSEs in doses above 8 mg/day. Zotepine can also cause EPSEs within the normal dosage range. Other atypicals are relatively free of EPSEs when used as antipsychotic monotherapy.

Risperidone
Potent 5-HT_2:D_2 antagonist. It was developed in line with the observation that ritanserin (a potent 5-HT_2 antagonist), when given in combination with conventional antipsychotics, was effective in treating the negative and affective symptoms of schizophrenia, and was the first of the new 'atypicals' to be marketed. In doses of less than 6 mg/day, it has few EPSEs and a low incidence of sedation. There is a potent first-dose hypotensive effect (due to α_1 block), so dosage titration is required. Serum prolactin is raised. A depot preparation may be available soon.

Olanzapine
Also a 5-HT_2:D_2 antagonist. It causes less postural hypotension but more sedation than risperidone. Serum prolactin is not raised. Olanzapine is usually very well tolerated, although weight gain can be problematic. Serum levels can be monitored as a guide to compliance or toxicity (there is no agreed therapeutic range). It is available as a soluble tablet that dissolves on contact with saliva.

Quetiapine
Low affinity for D_1, D_2 and 5-HT receptors and moderate affinity for adrenergic α_1 and α_2. Dosage titration is required (because of α_1 block). It has no effect on serum prolactin. Unlike risperidone or olanzapine, twice-daily dosing is required.

Amisulpride
Similar to sulpiride in that lower doses (300 mg/day or less) selectively block presynaptic dopamine receptors, leading to an increase in dopamine

transmission in the prefrontal cortex (the supposed site of the genesis of negative symptoms). At higher doses it blocks postsynaptic receptors and is relatively selective for limbic areas, translating clinically into a low potential for EPSEs. It is relatively free from sedation, anticholinergic side-effects and postural hypotension but is a particularly potent elevator of serum prolactin. The difference clinically between sulpiride and amisulpride is unclear.

Zotepine

Antagonist at 5-HT_{2a}, 5-HT_{2c}, D_1, D_2, D_3 and D_4 receptors, a potent inhibitor of noradrenaline (norepinephrine) reuptake, a potent H_1 antagonist (sedation) with some adrenergic α_1 block and possibly some activity at *N*-methyl D-aspartate (NMDA) receptors. It raises serum prolactin and is associated with a high incidence of seizures. Doses above 300 mg/day (frequently used, according to the available literature) and antipsychotic polypharmacy increase this risk.

Clozapine

Unique in two ways:

- It is more effective than other antipsychotics
- EPSEs are very rare (established tardive dyskinesia may even be reversed)

Robust studies have shown that two-thirds of patients who have failed to respond to other antipsychotics show meaningful gains if treated with clozapine for at least 1 year. Clozapine reduces positive symptoms, secondary negative symptoms, EPSEs and tardive dyskinesia, suicidality and aggression. The major drawback is the small risk of agranulocytosis, which can be fatal. Neutropenia occurs in 3% of patients and agranulocytosis in 0.8%. The risk of agranulocytosis is increased in Asians and the elderly and is greatest in the first 18 weeks of treatment.

Patients must be registered with the clozapine patient monitoring services (CPMS) and have blood taken before commencement of treatment and then weekly for the first 18 weeks, 2-weekly until 1 year and then 4-weekly if haematologically stable. The CPMS alerts the clinician to a green, amber or red alert result: these mean 'satisfactory', 'more samples are required' and 'withdraw the drug', respectively. If the drug is withdrawn, samples must be taken for a further 4 weeks to ensure recovery of the bone marrow.

OPTIMIZING CLOZAPINE TREATMENT

- Use as monotherapy if possible. If not, use haloperidol or droperidol during crossover
- Start with 12.5 mg at night (because of α_1 block). Increase gradually to 300–400 mg/day unless limited by side-effects
- If no response after several weeks, monitor trough serum level (before first dose of the day). This should be more than 0.35 mg/l
- If less than 0.35 mg/l and response poor, increase dose to produce a level above 0.35 mg/l. Assess over several weeks
- If still no/poor response, increase the dose to the maximum tolerated (up to 900 mg/day)

Remember

- Only 50% of responders do so in the first 6 weeks
- A clozapine withdrawal syndrome can occur, so in non-emergency situations clozapine should be stopped slowly

ADVERSE EFFECTS OF CLOZAPINE

- Sedation (dose-related, give larger/whole dose at night)
- Hypersalivation (try hyoscine or pirenzepine)
- Postural hypotension (use fludrocortisone in extreme cases)
- Seizures (occur in 5% of patients who receive more than 600 mg/day; sodium valproate is effective)
- Constipation (dietary advice and laxatives)
- Weight gain (difficult to manage)
- Nocturnal enuresis (oxybutynin or desmopressin may help)
- Tachycardia (β-blocker may be useful, ECG advised)
- Nausea
- Myocarditis, probably due to hypersensitivity

CLOZAPINE AND THE MENTAL HEALTH ACT 1983

Taking blood is not clearly covered under the Mental Health Act but as it is necessary to ensure the 'safe' treatment of a patient on clozapine, treatment under the Act is usually interpreted to include taking blood. No case has yet come to court but the assumption is that blood samples are a necessary part of the treatment. In view of the risks, it is always prudent to involve the family or next of kin in treatment decisions.

Benzodiazepines

Used as anxiolytics, hypnotics, muscle relaxants, anticonvulsants, for myoclonus and for sedation during short operative procedures. They are increasingly used in rapid tranquillization regimens and for short-term behavioural control in psychotic illness. Diazepam and chlordiazepoxide are standard treatments in the management of withdrawal symptoms associated with detoxification from alcohol.

Benzodiazepines exert their anxiolytic effect by potentiating the action of the inhibitory neurotransmitter γ-aminobutyric acid (GABA). Flumazenil also binds to the same molecular complex and reverses the action of benzodiazepines, although its half-life is shorter than many of the benzodiazepines.

Benzodiazepines should not be prescribed in the long term and only for specific disorders where they are of proven benefit. They are helpful as an adjunct in the treatment of acute psychoses and severe panic attacks. Where they are used for neurosis, a behavioural programme should be initiated and the short term nature of the pharmacological approach, mainly for crisis intervention, must be clearly established with the patient. For example, in the treatment of insomnia, the following must be considered:

- Is the underlying cause being treated, e.g. depression, breathing difficulties, pain, etc?
- Is substance misuse or diet a problem?

- Are other drugs being given at appropriate times, e.g. procyclidine in the early part of the day, sedative antipsychotics at night?
- Is the patient's expectation of sleep realistic? About 90% of adults sleep 6–9 hours each night. The need for sleep decreases with age and some of the elderly require less than 6 hours of sleep per night
- Avoid prescription for those with a history of alcohol or drug dependency, as dependency is likely
- Avoid prescription for those with personality disorder, especially of the dissocial type, because these drugs may disinhibit aggression

Remember, sleep hygiene should always be encouraged:

- Increase daily exercise
- Reduce daytime napping
- Reduce caffeine and alcohol consumption, especially in the evening
- Use anxiety management techniques

If benzodiazepines are used as hypnotics:

- Use the lowest effective dose
- Use intermittent dosing where possible
- Never prescribe for more than 4 weeks
- Discontinue slowly
- Be alert for rebound insomnia/withdrawal symptoms
- Advise patients of the interaction with alcohol
- In general, aim to use a low dose of a longer-acting preparation (drugs with shorter half-lives are most likely to cause dependency)
- Do not continue for more than 4 weeks

Several new non-benzodiazepine hypnotics are available (zopiclone, zolpidem and zaleplon). There is no evidence to support a lower dependence potential with these drugs.

Buspirone (a non-benzodiazepine), propranolol and SSRIs are alternative options in chronic anxiety states.

When used for behavioural disturbance in psychotic patients, the most commonly prescribed oral benzodiazepine is lorazepam (up to 4 mg four times a day in extreme disturbance). When the parenteral route is required, lorazepam (i.m.) and diazepam (i.v.) are most frequently used.

Table 11 Benzodiazepines

	Half-life (h)	Half-life of metabolite (h)	Approximate equivalent dose (mg)
Diazepam	20–50	40–200	10
Chlordiazepoxide	5–30	130	20
Lorazepam	10–20	Nil	2
Nitrazepam	28	Nil	20
Temazepam	8	12	20

SIDE-EFFECTS OF BENZODIAZEPINES

- Sedation, fatigue and apathy
- Ataxia, diplopia dysarthria and incoordination. Falls in the elderly
- Impaired memory, poor concentration and prolonged reaction times
- Paradoxical excitement and rage reactions
- Pseudohallucinations
- REM sleep suppression with rebound the following day
- Dependence, both psychological and physical. Post-withdrawal states can last many weeks or months
- Although there is little cardiovascular or respiratory depression, this may be potentiated by alcohol and other CNS depressants
- Rarely transient hypotension and apnoea
- Allergy is uncommon but thrombophlebitis after intravenous administration is accompanied by pain. Intra-arterial administration leads to spasm, ischaemia and possibly gangrene
- Note that some SSRIs inhibit benzodiazepine metabolism and hepatic or renal failure can contribute to the development of toxicity

Management of benzodiazepine withdrawal

The elderly with multiple physical health problems are especially at risk of becoming the new long-term users of benzodiazepines.

The Mental Health Foundation guidelines advocate a two-pronged approach: encouraging and managing withdrawal, and preventing new cases. Although there are good reasons for continuing prescriptions for patients who are long-term users of benzodiazepines, doctors may overestimate the problems. The more potent and shorter-acting benzodiazepines carry a greater risk of dependence.

In withdrawal states the following symptoms can occur:

- Irritability
- Severe anxiety and panic; depression
- Headache
- Insomnia
- Muscle and joint pains, and flu-like symptoms
- Tinnitus
- Fits
- Hypersensitivity to light and sound
- Depersonalization and derealization symptoms
- Visual and auditory hallucinations

MANAGING ACUTE WITHDRAWAL

- Change to longer-acting preparations (usually diazepam) before withdrawal
- If fits have occurred during previous withdrawals, hospital admission should be considered for the early stages
- Cognitive behavioural treatments should be considered
- Symptomatic treatment with a beta-blocker and antidepressant may be helpful but do not always allay the withdrawal symptoms

There is no agreed decrement that is suitable for all patients, although a reduction in dose of one-eighth every 2 weeks has been suggested as most suitable. It is best to titrate the dose of diazepam against emergent withdrawal symptoms. Withdrawal may take up to 16 weeks in uncomplicated cases but in some, symptoms may persist for many years.

Antidepressants

All antidepressants are equally effective. Side-effect profiles, drug interactions and safety in overdose vary markedly.

Antidepressants should be taken in a therapeutic dose for a minimum of 6 months after recovery (9 months in all) from a single episode of depression. Current guidelines indicate that antidepressant treatment should be continued for 2 years (or longer) if there have been two or more episodes of severe depression within 5 years.

All patients taking benzodiazepines should know that:

- The risk of recurrence of depressive illness is high and increases with each episode
- The risk of relapse is greatly reduced by taking antidepressants
- Antidepressants:
  - are effective
  - are not addictive
  - usually need to be taken for 10–14 days before therapeutic effects are manifest
  - do not lose their efficacy over time
  - are not known to cause long-term side-effects
  - need to be taken and continued at the full treatment dose for the duration of treatment
  - should not be stopped suddenly as this may lead to discontinuation symptoms. These include agitation, irritability, insomnia, movement disorders, vivid dreams, cognitive impairment, chills, myalgia, sweating, nausea, headaches, dizziness, electric-shock-like sensations. The greatest risk is with short-half-life drugs e.g. paroxetine, venlafaxine.

Tricyclic antidepressants

These are used in major depression, phobic anxiety states and other neuroses, enuresis, atypical facial pain and chronic pain.

Tricyclic drugs act by blocking amine (noradrenaline (norepinephrine), 5-HT (serotonin), dopamine) reuptake into presynaptic neurones after neuronal discharge. The clinical effect takes at least 10 days to become manifest, even although in animal studies the blockade of uptake is immediate. The postsynaptic receptor down-regulation in response to higher neurotransmitter concentrations in the synaptic cleft seems to have the same time course as the clinical effect. Tertiary amines undergo hepatic metabolism to produce secondary amine metabolites, which also are active antidepressants. The therapeutic dose for most tricyclics is at least 150 mg/day, a dose that is rarely reached in primary care. Dosage titration is required for all tricyclics at the start of treatment (because of adrenergic α_1 block).

Amitriptyline and dosulepin (dothiepin) are more sedating than imipramine.

Clomipramine is a potent 5-HT reuptake inhibitor and is useful in OCD and panic disorder as well as depression.

Lofepramine is a noradrenaline (norepinephrine) reuptake inhibitor that has a more favourable side-effect profile than the older tricyclics and is safer in overdose.

ADVERSE EFFECTS OF TRICYCLICS

- Sedation
- Seizures (dose-related)
- Headache
- Myoclonus, paraesthesias and other movement disorders
- Hypomania
- Increased appetite and weight gain
- Hyponatraemia
- Anticholinergic effects: blurred vision, dry mouth, constipation, paralytic ileus, hesitancy, urinary retention, impotence, delayed orgasm, sweating, aggravated glaucoma, acute confusion
- Cardiac effects: alpha blockade causes hypotension, sexual dysfunction. Palpitations, supraventricular tachyarrhythmias, AV block, bundle branch block, T wave and ST depression, prolonged PR, QRS and QT intervals on ECG
- Rare: cholestatic jaundice, vasculitis, dermatitis, blood dyscrasias
- Discontinuation symptoms on withdrawal of treatment

Monoamine oxidase inhibitors

Monoamine oxidase inhibitors (MAOIs) inhibit the action of monoamine oxidase, which metabolizes amine neurotransmitters in the nerve terminals after reuptake. They take 7–14 days to exert an antidepressant effect. MAOIs are used for atypical depressions and where other antidepressants have failed, and are especially useful where anxiety symptoms predominate.

Inhibitors of MAO type A inhibit the breakdown of 5-HT (serotonin) and noradrenaline, while inhibitors of MAO type B prevent dopamine breakdown (selective MAOB inhibitors, e.g. selegiline, are used in the treatment of Parkinson's disease).

Phenelzine and tranylcypromine are irreversible inhibitors of both MAOA and MAOB. Note that tranylcypromine is metabolized to amfetamine and is the exception to the rule that antidepressants are not addictive. It is due to be withdrawn from the market in 2001 and will only be available on a named patient basis.

Moclobemide is a reversible inhibitor of MAOA (meaning very low risk of interaction with tyramine-containing foods).

ADVERSE EFFECTS OF MAOIS

- Postural hypotension
- Headache
- Dry mouth, blurred vision and constipation
- Mania

- Weight gain
- Blood dyscrasias
- Hepatotoxicity
- Hyponatraemia
- Hypertensive crises due to food and drug interactions
- Food and drug interactions
- Dietary tyramine is metabolized by MAO. Therefore consumption of large quantities of tyramine in food (e.g. mature cheese, Chianti wine, pickled herrings) can lead to hypertensive crisis. The tyramine content of food varies substantially and is difficult to predict
- The concomitant use of other drugs that increase monoamine neurotransmission should also be avoided (e.g. tricyclics, SSRIs, pethidine, levodopa, sumatriptan and sympathomimetics such as ephedrine and phenylephrine). All food and drug interactions can occur for 2 weeks after the MAOI is discontinued. MAOI warning cards are available and these give detailed advice about which foods and drugs to avoid

Selective serotonin reuptake inhibitors

These drugs inhibit the reuptake of 5-HT (serotonin) into presynaptic neurones. They have a different side-effect profile from the tricyclics and are much safer in overdose. They are simple to use, in that dosage titration is not required in most patients (i.e. it is difficult to use subtherapeutic doses). They are especially helpful in patients with OCD or phobic anxiety states. Fluoxetine is also licensed for bulimia and premenstrual dysphoric disorder, and paroxetine for social phobia.

ADVERSE EFFECTS OF SSRIS

- Abdominal bloating, nausea, diarrhoea and dyspepsia
- Anorexia with weight loss
- Dry mouth
- Headaches
- Anxiety
- Sexual dysfunction, especially ejaculatory delay
- Movement disorders
- Serotonergic syndrome: hyperactivity, agitation, hyperthermia and tachycardia, especially if combined with tricyclics, MAOIs or L-tryptophan
- Insomnia
- Seizures
- Hyponatraemia
- Discontinuation syndrome: agitation, irritability, insomnia, movement disorders, vivid dreams, cognitive impairment, chills, myalgia, sweating, nausea, headaches, dizziness, electric-shock-like sensations
- Paroxetine has a short half-life and therefore a high incidence of discontinuation symptoms
- Citalopram is the most 5-HT-specific SSRI and has the least potential for interactions with other drugs
- Fluvoxamine commonly causes nausea and is rarely used

- Fluoxetine has a long half-life and is therefore least likely to lead to discontinuation syndrome. However, a long half-life means that a 3–4-day washout period must be allowed if switching to a tricyclic or another SSRI (2 weeks if switching to an MAOI). Fluoxetine is also a potent inhibitor of CYP2C, CYP2D6 and CYP3A4, causing increased plasma levels of phenytoin, warfarin, tricyclics, clozapine and benzodiazepines

Other antidepressants

- **VENLAFAXINE**
  5-HT and noradrenaline (norepinephrine) reuptake inhibitor (like amitriptyline but minimal effects on other transmitter pathways). Associated with serotonergic and adrenergic side-effects as well as increased BP in doses above 200 mg/day, and raised cholesterol
- **NEFAZODONE**
  5-HT reuptake inhibitor which also blocks postsynaptic 5-HT_2 and 5-HT_3 receptors. Associated with nausea, mild anticholinergic side-effects and postural hypotension, but less sexual dysfunction than SSRIs
- **MIRTAZAPINE**
  Blocks presynaptic α_2 receptors on both noradrenaline (norepinephrine) and 5-HT neurones, as well as postsynaptic 5-HT_2 and 5-HT_3 receptors. It is chemically related to mianserin. Sedative and causes weight gain but is associated with a low incidence of sexual dysfunction
- **REBOXETINE**
  Specific noradrenaline (norepinephrine) reuptake inhibitor that also blocks presynaptic α_2 receptors. Activating, must be given twice daily and not licensed for use in the elderly. Useful in patients who experience lethargy

Mood stabilizers

Lithium

Lithium is used in the prophylaxis of bipolar affective disorder and unipolar depression, as augmentation in refractory depression, to prevent self-mutilation in those with learning difficulties and as an anti-impulse agent in those with any of the impulse disorders. Lithium reduces the number and severity of relapses in bipolar disorder and may help prevent antidepressant-induced hypomania. Lithium may also be used in the treatment of acute mania but it is not sedative and takes around 2 weeks to exert an effect.

The mechanism of action remains elusive. It may involve regulation of Na^+/K^+ channel opening in neuronal membranes. Regulation of phosphatidylinositol messenger systems may also play an important part. Lithium is not metabolized and is renally excreted.

Therapeutic level monitoring is essential as high serum levels can lead to irreversible renal toxicity. For mania or prophylaxis, the therapeutic range is

0.6–1.0 mmol/l. For elderly patients, sodium-depleted patients or those with impaired renal function or CNS disease, or in order to augment antidepressants, lower levels (0.4–0.8 mmol/l) may suffice.

Lithium treatment must be monitored by means of blood tests at least every 6 months once steady plasma level has been obtained.

- Serum lithium level, measured at least 5 days after a dosage change (steady state achieved) and 12 hours after the last dose
- Urea and electrolytes
- Thyroid function tests (and consider antithyroid antibodies in middle-aged women, for whom risk of hypothyroidism is greatest)
- ECG (before commencing treatment)

All patients taking lithium should know:

- That lithium is a long-term treatment (there is a high rate of manic relapse after lithium is discontinued)
- That it is important to take the prescribed dose at the same time every day
- That regular blood tests are required, and why
- That they should consider interactions with any new medication (diuretics, NSAIDs and angiotensin-converting enzyme inhibitors all raise lithium levels)
- That dehydration and high salt diet can lead to toxicity
- How to recognize the symptoms of lithium toxicity (blurred vision, drowsiness, confusion, palpitations) and what to do about them.

ADVERSE EFFECTS OF LITHIUM – DOSE-DEPENDENT

- Fine tremor (especially affecting the hands)
- Ataxia
- Dysarthria
- Drowsiness
- Weakness
- Polyuria and thirst, diarrhoea
- Nystagmus
- Spasticity and hyper-reflexia
- Nausea and vomiting, confusion, coma, dehydration, death (if dose more than 4 mmol/l)

ADVERSE EFFECTS OF LITHIUM – DOSE-INDEPENDENT

- Hypothyroidism
- Thirst and polyuria due to nephrogenic diabetes insipidus
- Cardiac conduction delays and arrhythmias
- Leukopenia
- Weight gain
- Peripheral oedema
- Skin conditions such as psoriasis can be exacerbated
- Teratogenesis: if given in first trimester can cause Ebstein's congenital anomaly (low-set tricuspid valve – 1:1000 but relative risk 20)
- Lithium is secreted in breast milk (therefore best avoided in breast-feeding mothers)

Carbamazepine

Carbamazepine is an anticonvulsant used for grand mal epilepsy and focal seizures. It is also used in trigeminal neuralgia, phantom limb pain and alcohol withdrawal. Anticonvulsants have a truly antimanic effect and are used when lithium and/or neuroleptics have been unsuccessful. Carbamazepine is most effective in rapid-cycling patients, who usually do not respond to lithium treatment. Combination therapy may be necessary in such patients.

Clinical effects can take 2 weeks to develop. Serum levels of 8–12 mmol/l are optimal, although some patients will respond at lower levels. Carbamazepine is an enzyme inducer. Its half-life is 30 hours but on chronic dosing is 12 hours. It has weak antidepressant properties and has a similar structure to tricyclic antidepressants. A washout period is needed before administration after an MAOI.

- **ADVERSE EFFECTS OF CARBAMAZEPINE**
  - Drowsiness
  - Ataxia
  - Diplopia
  - Dysarthria
  - Aplastic anaemia (1:20 000) and agranulocytosis (warn patients about fever and obtain pretreatment and regular full blood counts)
  - Hypersensitivity, including rashes
  - Inappropriate antidiuretic hormone syndrome, leading to hyponatraemia
  - Raised alkaline phosphatase and γ-glutamyl transferase indicate hypersensitivity and possible hepatitis. Stop treatment
  - Enzyme inducer. Can render oral contraceptive and other anticonvulsants ineffective (can also cause anticonvulsant toxicity)
  - Serum levels raised by cimetidine, calcium channel blockers, erythromycin, fluoxetine and dextropropoxyphene
  - Neurotoxic reactions, although uncommon, can occur when used with lithium

Other mood stabilizers

- **SODIUM VALPROATE**
  Frequently used, although not licensed for this purpose in the UK. At least 1000 mg/day is normally required, giving a trough level of at least 50 μg/l. Side-effects include nausea, lethargy, confusion, weight gain, peripheral oedema, hair loss, blood dyscrasias, pancreatitis and hepatic damage (rare)
- There is some evidence that **lamotrigine**, **gabapentin**, **topiramate** and **phenytoin** may also have mood stabilizing properties

ELECTROCONVULSIVE THERAPY

Indications for ECT treatment include:

- Major depression with psychosis
- Major depression not responding to drug treatment
- Major depression where a quick response is essential (severe weight loss or stupor)
- Puerperal psychosis
- Catatonic schizophrenia
- Acute mania that does not respond to other interventions.

Studies demonstrate that, despite a big placebo effect, ECT is effective. The onset of the response is quicker than when drug treatment is used. Bilateral treatment, although better, produces more post-ECT confusion than unilateral treatment. The latter should only be used if there is severe post-ECT confusion and then is administered to the non-dominant side. Between four and six treatments are usually necessary for a minimal response to be seen. A maximum of 12 treatments is usual. ECT is optimally given on two or three occasions a week; progress should be reviewed weekly and notes made about the seizure type, duration, anaesthetic agents and any complications. If a fit does not visibly occur, check with the anaesthetist that the patient is adequately sedated, and try again at a higher voltage. If this fails do not try for a third time. Note that fit threshold increases as a treatment proceeds. Higher currents may need to be delivered if a fit does not occur or the duration of the fit for any one current setting is falling.

In order to minimize side-effects, the Royal College of Psychiatrists recommends both stimulus dosing and EEG monitoring. When stimulus dosing is used, the seizure threshold is determined during the first treatment session and the voltage is increased with each subsequent session. EEG monitoring allows cerebral seizure activity to monitored. It has been shown that some individuals experience prolonged seizures, which are not manifest in tonic–clonic movements. Such seizures may be associated with subsequent memory loss and confusion. Generalized seizures lasting for more than 60 s should be terminated by means of intravenous diazepam.

A sphygmomanometer cuff to prevent the passage of muscle relaxant into the forearm may be used to examine visually the onset and termination of a seizure and hence the duration, which should be at least 20–25 s. There is an increase in cerebral blood flow by up to 200%. An initial bradycardia is followed by a sudden tachycardia; the heart rate then falls to just below the resting rate and then there is sustained slight tachycardia for minutes. With muscle relaxants the blood pressure does not rise to extremes but the systolic pressure can still occasionally reach 200 mmHg.

The exact therapeutic component remains elusive. During the procedure, neurochemical changes include elevated levels of tryptophan, raised monoamine oxidase activity and increased blood–brain barrier permeability. Prolactin is raised 20 min after a seizure; this rise attenuates as treatment proceeds but is sometimes measured to ensure that a seizure took place. In at least one study, it has been demonstrated that elevation of oxytocin-related neurophysin after ECT correlates with improvement. There is increased cortisol and ACTH release but growth hormone and TSH are not usually affected. The EEG shows a build-up of diffuse, irregular, low-frequency activity, with delta and some theta activity. There is greater REM sleep, reduced REM latency and a reduction in total sleep time.

Table 12 Neurotransmitter effects of electroconvulsive therapy and antidepressants

Receptor	ECT	Antidepressants
5-HT_1	Decreased	Decreased
5-HT_2	Increased	Decreased
Dopamine	No change	No change
γ-aminobutyric acid	Increased	Increased
β-adrenergic	Decreased	Decreased
α_2-adrenergic	Decreased	Decreased
α_1-adrenergic	No change	No change

CONTRAINDICATIONS TO ECT

- Raised intracranial pressure
- Recent cerebrovascular haemorrhage
- Cerebral or aortic aneurysm
- Myocardial infarction in previous three months
- Acute chest infections and other contraindications for general anaesthesia

BEFORE ADMINISTERING ECT

- Check urea and electrolytes
- Carry out thorough physical examination to exclude the possibility of cardiac and chest disease
- Record pulse and blood pressure
- Consider ECG and chest X-ray if elderly or physically ill
- Obtain CT if possibility of space-occupying lesion

The patient should be fasted as for any general anaesthetic (at least 6 h) and should be well hydrated (better fits). All patients (especially day patients) should specifically be asked about the last time they ate. Preoxygenation (hyperventilation) by the anaesthetist also facilitates seizure activity. Premedication with anticholinergics has traditionally been administered but is now less often used. Other medications such as anticonvulsants, benzodiazepines and tryptophan are likely to increase the fit threshold.

Handedness should be identified if unilateral placement is considered necessary. In right-handed people, the left hemisphere is nearly always dominant, whereas in left-handed people it is only dominant in 25–50% of cases.

Training in electrode placement, types of machine and postseizure management should be provided before anyone attempts to apply the treatment. In some centres, ambulatory ECG monitoring and pulse oximetry are the norm. The Royal College of Psychiatrists' guidelines advise that recovery and waiting rooms should be available, separate from the room in which the treatment takes place. A nurse should attend each patient while they recover from the anaesthetic.

Success rates of over 70–80% with ECT, 60–70% with antidepressants and 20–30% with placebo have been demonstrated. Relapse rates do not differ. Maintenance treatment with antidepressants is advised as patients may relapse after a successful trial of ECT.

ADVERSE EFFECTS OF ECT

- Confusion
- Headache
- Amnesia (both retrograde and anterograde, receding within 3 months of the treatment)
- Muscle pain
- Burns
- Urinary incontinence
- Broken teeth
- Vertebral fracture
- Cardiac arrhythmias
- Myocardial infarction
- Cerebral haemorrhage
- Aspiration pneumonia
- Pulmonary embolus

Traumatic injuries are far less common now because of the use of muscle relaxants and brief anaesthesia with an anaesthetist present. Lasting memory impairment is unlikely; in those complaining of persistent memory problems it seems that these are often due to persistent depressive symptoms.

PSYCHOSURGERY

About 20–30 operations are performed annually in two centres in the UK.

Most operations are stereotactic subcaudate tractotomies (SSTs, all at the Geoffrey Knight Unit, Brook General Hospital), although some are stereotactic limbic leukotomies (SLLs, mostly at Atkinson Morley). Amygdalotomy is performed to treat pathological aggression; SST for depression, OCD and, occasionally, treatment-resistant anxiety symptoms. SLL is usually carried out for OCD and disorders involving refractory obsessive symptoms. The procedure has now been considerably refined: radioactive yttrium seeds are located at the target site using a stereotactic frame.

Psychosurgery is only performed if the patient has been exposed to all other possible treatments for the optimal lengths of time and drug doses. Assessment involves a reappraisal of the symptoms, history, neurological state and review of the treatments tried and their potential efficacy. If all treatments have not been exhausted then these are attempted prior to operative treatment. Thus, a series of pharmacological treatments at high dose and with the necessary adjunctive therapies are attempted. For severe depression, this amounts to high-dose clomipramine with lithium and L-tryptophan on a named-patient basis, possibly adding triiodothyronine and an adequate trial of ECT.

Severe dementia, personality disorders and severe physical illness that makes the anaesthetic procedure hazardous are contraindications to psychosurgery. Assessment is made by a neurosurgeon and a psychiatrist with special knowledge of this field.

Some clinicians argue that there is no place for such a treatment in modern practice; others argue that it is necessary in severe intractable disorders where other approaches have failed and where there is severe distress and the suicide risk is high. Improvement rates with SST are approximately 70% for depression and 50–60% for anxiety states, including OCD. Limbic leukotomy is thought to be better for OCD, with response rates of over 80%. The absence of control groups (which would pose an ethical dilemma) makes a rigorous assessment difficult but, in view of the refractory nature of the disorders, outcomes can be compared using cases as their own controls. More work needs to be done on the social and psychological outcomes of patients undergoing this treatment.

All patients undergoing the procedure must be able to give informed consent. If they cannot (as in the case of some of the most severely ill), the Mental Health Act does not allow such treatment to be given. Two independent doctors must agree that the patient is able to give consent.

ADVERSE EFFECTS OF PSYCHOSURGERY

- Incontinence
- Apathy
- Seizures
- Memory impairment
- Personality change (very rare)
- Weight gain (very rare)
- Disinhibition
- Death (1:1200)

PSYCHOLOGICAL TREATMENTS

Psychological treatments are considered essential by most users of psychiatric services. In recent years, there has been a rapid expansion in the employment of counsellors by GPs and in the forms of psychological treatment offered in both primary and secondary care settings. The requirements of the Royal College of Psychiatrists reflect this, stating that trainees must gain experience in a number of different models of psychological intervention. In considering what psychological treatment might be most appropriate for a patient, both the form of treatment and the context (individual, couple, family or group) are important.

FORMS OF PSYCHOLOGICAL TREATMENT

Forms of psychological treatment tend to lie on a continuum of both length of treatment and depth of work. The divisions shown below are therefore somewhat arbitrary, and overlap occurs. There is no suggestion that one form of treatment is better than another: each patient and set of circumstances needs to be carefully assessed.

Psychoeducation

This form of psychological treatment is appropriate, possibly essential, in any form of mental illness. It is a process that involves two stages. Firstly, a healthcare professional, as the expert on psychopathology and treatment, informs the patient, and their carers and support network, about the illness with which they have been diagnosed. This will involve explaining symptoms, illness patterns, treatment options, preventative measures and prognosis. Secondly, the patient, as the expert on their unique experience of the illness, needs to be given time to inform the professionals about their symptoms, beliefs about causation, factors that improve or worsen symptoms, feelings, fears and the effect of the illness on their daily functioning.

This bidirectional flow of information means that a management plan can be negotiated that is individually tailored, acceptable to the patient and offers optimal chances of amelioration of, or recovery from, symptoms. The plan will pay particular attention to enabling the patient to recognize warning signs of deterioration or relapse, and encouraging strategies for coping with the illness and obtaining appropriate support when required.

Psychoeducation is particularly important in chronic relapsing mental illnesses such as schizophrenia, where it may (for example) persuade a reluctant patient to comply with long-term medication. It may also enable families to develop realistic expectations and to support professionals in their advised management plan. It may also prevent the development of anxiety and high emotional expression, thus contributing to a reduction in relapses.

Crisis intervention

A crisis has been described as 'any problem that seems insurmountable and beyond normal coping mechanisms'. Continuing inability to resolve a crisis can lead to exhaustion and progressive deterioration in mental wellbeing and social functioning. A person can be helped through a crisis by informal or professional support. Research has shown the protective value of a trusted friend or confidante in relapsing depression. Mental health professionals, those who work in casualty departments and general practice staff can be trained in the basic techniques of crisis intervention, which may need to be offered on one occasion or to be formalized into a short course of focused psychological treatment.

Assessment of a person in crisis should take account of any past history of mental illness, perceived problems and any steps already taken to alleviate the situation. It will also need to include details of secondary problems, the level of support available to the person in crisis and details of how the person has coped in the past. Depending on the level of functioning, the client in crisis may only require an empathic ear, support in decision-making and help in planning a stepwise strategy to deal with the crisis. Crisis intervention can also be directive, and advice may be given.

Where functioning is severely affected, it may be necessary for a professional or mental health team to temporarily take control. This may enable the client to recuperate sufficiently to begin to engage in the process of forming more successful coping strategies to enable resolution themselves.

Often, crisis intervention requires a high initial input for a relatively short period. A keyworker may need to network with other agencies and often needs to meet with a client's family and support network. It may be necessary for a client to move out of a very stressful situation, and a psychiatric admission may be appropriate.

Specific crisis intervention agencies exist to help with such problems as alcohol or drug relapse, and for victims of violent or sexual incidents. Such agencies hold expert knowledge of both appropriate interventions and available services.

Counselling

Counselling is usually offered by non-medical staff. Counselling is generally non-directive, non-judgemental, empathic, supportive and enables clients to cope more effectively with their current life circumstances or inner state. Clients find it helpful to air their problems, ventilate their feelings and feel heard and held. They may gain a new perspective on their difficulties and discover new resources with which they can deal with them. It can be useful as a form of support at times of traumatic life events in the psychologically well, and can also offer help to those with chronic conditions in terms of increasing coping abilities.

Many different models of counselling exist. Counsellors in the UK are usually accredited through the British Association for Counselling, which requires a code of ethics and practice, and training by a recognized organization. Regular supervision is also important.

Routes to counselling are numerous. Many GPs now employ counsellors, counselling training organizations offer low-cost counselling, and private counsellors advertise and are listed on professional registers. Many social workers and nurses have additional counselling qualifications, and specialist counsellors are employed by voluntary organizations, rehabilitation centres, etc. When clients request 'talking treatment', they are generally referring to counselling.

Counselling can be at many different levels. A short course of supportive sessions could be appropriate for anyone from a usually well but recently bereaved professional person to the carer of someone with a major disability, or someone with a long-term mental illness experiencing particular worries. Supportive counselling aims to offer reassurance, facilitate understanding and enable a client to function more effectively. It offers very limited opportunities for cognitive restructuring, unlike insight-oriented therapies such as psychoanalysis.

Counselling can also be more insight-oriented and work at deeper levels. In this format, clients would need to show a degree of psychological mindedness, a willingness to look at their own agency in negative situations and a desire for positive change. Such work, by its nature, tends to take longer. It would not be recommended for borderline or psychotic patients. Counsellors in general practice may only be able to work in a time-limited fashion and potential clients often need to seek private help or to obtain help from a specialist mental health team.

A referral to a counsellor should consider the counsellor's qualifications and level of supervision, as well as the length of contract he/she would be willing to offer.

Psychodynamic psychotherapy

In psychodynamic psychotherapy, the relationship between client and therapist is central to treatment. Within this context, psychological defences can be confronted, the past can be recalled and understood, interpersonal dynamics can be explored, regression can take place, unconscious phenomena can be interpreted and conflicts can be acted out and resolved. Psychotherapy aims to enable the client to bring about both outer and inner change.

Psychotherapists do not need to be medically qualified in the UK. As in counselling, many models of theory, practice and training exist and therapists can practise privately or be employed by health-care providers. Psychotherapy departments linked to psychiatric departments often offer an assessment service, both to assess the suitability of a referred client for psychotherapy and to determine which model and mode of delivery would be most appropriate.

Brief focused (psychodynamic) psychotherapy

This form of psychotherapy is currently gaining popularity in the UK, as research shows positive results in a number of different mental health problems. This treatment appeals to both clients, who understandably seek rapid results, and purchasers of services, who seek efficient, cost-effective, time-limited interventions. The principles behind brief focused therapy are that the therapist works in a psychodynamically informed way, that sessions are geared towards insight into current problems and their links with past experiences and personality patterns, and that there is a high level of intervention from the therapist. Homework tasks may be set. To be suitable, clients need to have circumscribed difficulties, a high level of motivation for change and a capacity for self-reflection. Contracts are often established for six sessions at a time, with an average of 25–30 weekly 1-hour sessions bringing improvement in a number of the neuroses, PTSD and other disorders.

Insight-oriented/exploratory psychodynamic psychotherapy

Within the therapeutic relationship, the unconscious is explored. Patients are offered regular, time-delineated sessions in a consistent setting. The therapist remains strictly neutral, does not offer advice and encourages free association. The patient's resistance and defence mechanisms are challenged, confronted and modified. Transference is fostered, revealed and interpreted, enabling re-enactment and remembering of early formative experiences. Dreams and fantasies are interpreted. Some models of psychotherapy use specific techniques to access the unconscious such as guided imagery and symbolic representation. Insights gained enable patients to develop a more whole view of themselves and their relationships with others, so that choices can be made about discarding outmoded ways of thinking and behaving and developing better ways of functioning.

Suitability for specialist psychotherapy entails a high level of motivation and commitment, a desire to learn more about oneself, psychological mindedness (sensing links between current difficulties and past traumas, for example), the capacity to enter into a relationship with a therapist and use this fully, an ability to tolerate anxiety, the capacity to be objective and the ability to respond to interpretations. Unsuitability would encompass psychotic or borderline psychopathology (except when treated by experienced and often medically trained therapists), serious impulsive or risk-taking behaviour and those seeking gratification from the therapeutic relationship rather than insight and change.

Within the NHS, psychotherapy is usually offered once weekly, or twice weekly in exceptional circumstances, and usually for a time-limited period, typically of 9–12 months. Consultant psychotherapists offer both an assessment and supervision service to maximize the number of patients who can be appropriately placed and treated. Either individual or group psychotherapy may be offered.

Psychoanalysis

Full psychoanalysis involves five-times-weekly analytic psychotherapy. The patient usually reclines on a couch, with the analyst out of view, and is invited to embark on free association. This intensive psychotherapeutic treatment enables a full exploration of the unconscious and cognitive and behavioural restructuring. It is a feasible and appropriate treatment option for only a small number of patients but the experience is the core training of most medically qualified psychotherapists.

Therapists may have been trained in a number of different theoretical models, a full description of which is beyond the scope of this handbook. In brief, Sigmund Freud developed the technique of free association and the concepts of transference, the Oedipus complex and ego splitting. Carl Jung developed the field of analytical psychology with the concepts of the personal and collective unconscious and archetypes, and viewed treatment as a process of individuation. Melanie Klein developed the field of child analysis and the theories of primitive defence mechanisms, the paranoid–schizoid and depressive positions, and the concept of identification with idealized internal objects. Anna Freud also developed child analysis and developmental theories and elaborated on defence mechanisms. John Bowlby developed attachment theory and Winnicott the concept of object relations and the use of transitional objects. Fritz Perls developed gestalt therapy with the use of active therapeutic techniques and Carl Rogers developed client-centred therapy. For more details on these and other theoretical models the reader is advised to consult a basic psychotherapy textbook.

An assessment of a potential client may reveal a preference or aptitude for a therapist trained in a particular model.

Behavioural therapy

Behavioural treatments are practical, problem-oriented and empirically based. Treatment aims to change dysfunctional behaviours. The therapist explores with the patient the antecedents of the behaviours, full details of the behaviours themselves and their consequences, and alternative behaviours are advised to break a maladaptive pattern. Behaviours are arranged in a graded hierarchy, with an agenda set to treat problem areas in a stepwise fashion so that gains can be seen by patients and carers and self-esteem and motivation remain high. Behavioural treatments are used to treat a number of the neuroses, in sexual dysfunction, and to bring about behavioural change in childhood disorders such as conduct disorder and hyperactivity and in children and adults with learning difficulties and challenging behaviours. Behavioural therapy is also used as an adjunct to other treatments in chronic psychoses and affective disorders. It is most often combined with cognitive therapy.

Behavioural treatments might range from advising a stepwise increase in activity in a chronically depressed person, through techniques for remembering to take medication in dementia, which could be offered by a GP or community nurse, to complex interventions delivered by trained behavioural therapists.

Some specific techniques are used in different disorders. Systematic desensitization and exposure is employed to treat phobias, operant conditioning or the use of rewards for desired behaviour (e.g. a star chart) in childhood disorders such as enuresis, and response prevention to treat obsessions. Some behaviourally based treatment packages, such as relaxation techniques and social skills training, can be useful in a broad range of psychiatric illnesses. Behavioural techniques can be learned in a one-to-one therapeutic relationship, in a group or within the dynamic of a couple or family, depending on the presenting problem.

Cognitive therapy

This is another form of problem-oriented psychological treatment. It is often used in conjunction with behavioural techniques (cognitive behavioural therapy) or with insight-oriented work (cognitive analytical therapy). It can be used as an alternative to pharmacological treatment (e.g. in depression) or as an adjunct to other treatments. In a contracted series of sessions, patients are taught a set of problem-solving techniques that enable them to gain control over their symptoms.

The principles behind cognitive therapy are that an individual's behavioural and emotional responses will be shaped by their interpretation and evaluation of information from the environment; that the processing of this information is disordered in psychological disturbance and manifests as irrational beliefs; and that patients can learn to identify and change this bias in information processing, resulting in symptomatic improvement.

Cognitive therapy was developed by Aaron Beck and colleagues in Philadelphia. There are specific cognitive models for depression, anxiety and other disorders. In depression, the cognitive triad is said to be a negative view of the self, the world and the future, and the depressed person experiences frequent negative automatic thoughts. There is often a core belief that the patient is worthless and that living is pointless. Such negative thoughts deepen depression and lead to behavioural manifestations of low activity, social withdrawal and poor coping abilities. In anxiety there is an overestimation of threat and an underestimation of coping and support factors. Patients view themselves as vulnerable, the world as dangerous and the future as unpredictable. In panic disorder there is a catastrophic misinterpretation of bodily sensations.

There are often underlying assumptions that predispose patients to emotional disturbance, which may have arisen early in life and which act as rules for living (e.g. 'If I am not a high achiever no-one will like me'). Critical events later in life can activate these assumptions (or schemata), leading to cognitive disturbances. Cognitive therapy aims to break into the vicious circles of maladaptive thinking and subsequent pathological behaviours.

The cognitive therapist and patient need to negotiate a collaborative working alliance. An assessment will be made of the presenting problems and areas of life that have been affected. These will be clarified in detail and the patient's motivations for change and reinforcements for stasis will be examined. The model of working is explained, which will include an explanation of the need for the patient to learn and work at new strategies for coping with and ultimately resolving symptoms. Some patients are unable to work with the model, if they believe that the therapist should cure them rather than that they must learn self-help mechanisms. A clear agenda and targets will be set, homework may be given and a series of sessions will be contracted. Family and carers may become involved as therapeutic allies, particularly if behavioural work is undertaken simultaneously. The therapist is quite directive, and offers encouragement.

Specific techniques will be taught that revolve around becoming more conscious of automatic and distorted cognitions and then learning strategies for changing them. These include distraction techniques, thought stopping and challenging irrational beliefs.

Cognitive, or cognitive behavioural, therapy is of proven value in depression, generalized anxiety, specific phobias, obsessional ruminations, panic disorder and chronic pain. It is being used more widely and successes have been reported in chronic fatigue syndrome and eating disorders. It can be used as an adjunct to pharmaceuticals, with an additive effect. There is also growing evidence that cognitive behavioural therapy is effective in controlling otherwise treatment-resistant psychotic symptoms, including hallucinations and delusions.

Like brief focused therapy, cognitive behavioural therapy appeals to purchasers of mental health care because it is time-limited and relatively inexpensive. Some GPs are purchasing specific sessions of therapy time. Therapists come from a variety of backgrounds, principally psychology.

CONTEXT OF PSYCHOLOGICAL TREATMENT

It is important to decide whether a patient should receive psychological treatment as an individual, within a group, with a marital or other partner, or within the context of the family. Factors that will influence this decision are the patient's presenting problem, their preference and the level of available resources. Individual therapy is not necessarily more expensive, especially in problem-focused treatments such as cognitive behavioural therapy, given the intensive level of therapeutic input.

Group therapy

This was first used by physicians at the turn of the century for support and teaching. Group psychotherapy was first described around 1920 by Moreno, who developed the practice of psychodrama for the re-enactment of early experiences, using the group as cast and audience. Group therapeutic factors have been described by Foulkes, Bion and Yalom. In essence, a group becomes a microcosm in which the group member can be confronted with the effects of their behaviour on others, where the individual receives support and challenge, and where the group provides a safe context in which to experiment with change. It is also possible to learn from the experiences and mistakes of others. Additionally, the group is often a cathartic forum and social skills can be gained. Groups can be psychodynamic in orientation, self-help groups or geared towards behavioural changes (e.g. social skills training) and can extend to the level of therapeutic communities.

Good candidates for group therapy are those who volunteer for a group rather than being coerced under pressure and who have good verbal and conceptual skills. They should have a concern with relationships or problems that can be focused in this way, be able to attend at a regular time (often for a longer time period than for individual work) and not be openly contemptuous.

The group will need to set its own boundaries regarding confidentiality and other matters such as acceptable lateness, missed sessions, sexual tensions, etc. The facilitator's role is to manage the boundaries and anxieties, to interpret, to encourage interactions, to discourage factors impeding the group's progress and to make use of what the group brings out.

Couple therapy

This is obviously of particular relevance when the presenting problem lies within the couple dynamic. However, couple therapy can also be useful if one partner has a particular psychiatric illness in that the 'well' partner can be co-opted as an adjunctive therapist; and also where a therapist feels that some work may need to be done as a couple to strengthen the relationship before one partner moves on to deeper individual therapy, which could involve remembering early traumas (e.g. sexual dysfunction in a marriage that a wife believes is due to her prior history of childhood sexual abuse). Couple therapy enables the exploration of differing expectations, communication patterns and goals. Aims should be specific and attainable and there should be a willingness to accept greater flexibility and changes in roles and responsibilities and to look for practical coping skills and solutions.

Family therapy

This is the accepted mode of service delivery in child and adolescent psychiatry. In some countries, such as Australia, many adult psychiatric illnesses are also treated in a family context. In family therapy the family, rather than one individual member, is viewed as the disturbed unit. Often a team of therapists works together, with a male and female therapist in the room with the family and others behind a screen or on video–audio link. Firstly, a family is encouraged to come together to engage, and the views of different family members are sought on current problems. Agreement needs to be reached on aims and expectations of therapy and on realistic goals. The family will be encouraged to improve communication, find new ways of resolving conflicts and focus on interactions. Specific interventions will be used, which may be behavioural, educational or interpretative. Interventions may focus on the power balance within a family, control mechanisms and distortions, and aim to change dysfunctional patterns.

The main theoretical models of family therapy are structural family therapy (Minuchin), systemic or Milan family therapy and strategic therapy (Haley). In all of these the role of the therapist will include encouraging family members to talk to one another rather than to the therapist, taking nothing for granted but exploring and elaborating and circular questioning. The structural family therapist will encourage enactment, reframing and changing the balance of power. A systemic therapist will look at inflexibilities, family rules and beliefs, and recurring dysfunctional patterns. A strategic therapist might view the presenting problem as a metaphor for an inflexible pattern of interaction and communication.

Although conjoint working has been described (seeing the whole family together) there are times when a collateral way of working (different therapists seeing different family members) is more appropriate. This might be particularly useful in some stages of abuse work.

Psychotherapy across cultures

There has been great concern recently that members of ethnic minorities have difficulty in gaining access to psychotherapy services, and that such services are not culturally sensitive. Transference phenomena are likely to be problematic whenever the cultural backgrounds of therapist and patient are very dissimilar. Nafsiyat, an intercultural psychotherapy centre, has practised intercultural therapy for many years with success. The centre deliberately set itself against ethnic matching except where issues of language made it unavoidable. Many black organizations still suspect, and say, that black experience cannot be understood unless the therapist has first-hand experience of being black. For example, a black patient's experience of racism may not be recognized by a non-black therapist as having had such a dramatic impact.

Further, Western therapists and psychiatrists are often confused as to which is the better approach. Finite resources exclude the possibility of routinely matching client and therapist by ethnicity, yet there may be instances in which racial matching is necessary. Should the client's own preference be taken into account? Certainly there are cases where a person might wish for therapy in English despite it being their second language; similarly, patients may refuse to see a therapist from the same ethnic group or culture for disclosure of acts or events that are, according to their culture, taboo.

All societies have some form of schema for distinguishing between desired and undesired states of being. They all have recognized and culturally sanctioned ways of returning an individual to a state of health. The patient's desired modality of treatment must therefore be identified, and it must be explained whether this can be offered or not, or indeed why culturally sanctioned treatments have failed. Furthermore, assumptions cannot be made that the patient has understood the purpose of therapy. A careful explanation needs to be given at the outset about the structure of the therapy on offer and why it *might* be of help to them.

One would expect the language in which therapy is undertaken not to impact on the theoretical model used; one must bear in mind, however, that psychotherapy packaged as it is in the West is ethnically slanted regardless of the ethnic origin of the therapist. That is not the same as saying that a black person is unable to use it, just that they have not previously had the opportunity. The requirement is therefore to take as much time as is necessary at the assessment stage to ensure that the therapist has fully understood the patient and their wishes and that the patient understands what is available, what demands that may entail and indeed how long they might attend for.

SOCIAL TREATMENTS

Social treatments need to be individually tailored, on the basis of need, and should not be geared solely towards the patient. Often, interventions aimed at carers, such as easing an application for attendance allowance or putting the carer in touch with a support group, enable patients to function well in the community.

UNDERLYING CONCEPTS

Understanding the role of the patient's social context within their illness

The psychiatrist or mental health team should obtain a social history, which gives clues to predisposing, precipitating and perpetuating factors in the patient's illness (e.g. predisposing – immigrant family seeking asylum; precipitating – stress over Home Office hearing; perpetuating – temporary crowded housing, financial worries, poor English) before a social treatment plan can be formulated.

Transcultural issues

A patient's illness, and a relevant management plan, should take account of transcultural factors. Beliefs about mental health, symptom patterns and presentation to services are all modified by the patient's cultural background, as are appropriate interventions. In particular, a mental health team will need to have a supply of leaflets printed in languages reflecting the ethnic mix of the local population. Access to non-family-member translators is important and the team will need to be aware of specific local facilities for those of different cultural backgrounds. Sex and ethnicity of the allocated keyworker may be important in engaging a patient.

Multidisciplinary working

Psychiatrists rarely have a thorough working knowledge of (for example) local libraries, reductions in leisure centre entrance fees for the unemployed and evening classes. Other members of the multidisciplinary team may have more expertise in social treatments. Social treatments often need to be presented in a stepwise fashion, and a keyworker who can act as a coordinator for a long-term plan is essential. Keyworkers need to develop particular skills in negotiating interagency cooperation if a patient is to benefit fully from social interventions.

Normalization

Social treatments should aim to restore a patient to as normal a role within society as is possible. To this end, social treatments aim at increasing self-esteem and obtaining a sense of mastery. Obviously, interventions that help a patient to gain skills, rather than providing others to perform tasks for them, are more beneficial.

Taking account of the patient's beliefs about their social context

Patients usually have strong opinions about which social factors cause them most stress and bring on relapses, and those that keep them healthy. Social treatments cannot be prescribed – they need to be negotiated with a patient. If patients do not see themselves as isolated they will not want to attend day centres. Such treatments need to make the most of a patient's motivating factors.

Treatment within society

Social treatments cannot be delivered solely at a team base. Work may need to be done within the patient's home with their family or support network. The patient may need support from a team worker to attend a class, or visit housing options. A team also needs to hold a database of local facilities – sectorization aids the process of accumulating such knowledge.

SPECIFIC SOCIAL NEEDS

Inadequate housing

This is often a cause of major stress, particularly in deprived inner city areas. Housing may be inadequate because it is temporary (provoking anxiety), in poor repair (leading to high heating bills, unsanitary conditions, etc.) or inappropriate (within a family with high expressed emotion, unsupported, pets not allowed, unsuitable for disabled, area of high racial tension, etc.). Improving a patient's housing may involve simply making a phone-call to get a boiler fixed; informing a council or housing association tenant that they have a named housing support worker; or tracking down a maintenance department or landlord. Helping a patient with rehousing will involve an assessment of need, particularly for the level of support required (24-hour staffed, day-only cover, warden available, group home, independent living). Patients with psychiatric illnesses are entitled to priority in housing allocation. Some areas have housing options available under health authority or specific mental health charity control.

Financial problems

Under community care guidelines, individuals are entitled to a needs assessment, which will involve financial review. Patients may be entitled to rebates or additional benefits (e.g. disability living allowance, grants to assist those leaving hospital). Input may be required from a debt counsellor, or training in budgeting may be needed (e.g. regular purchase of TV licence and utilities stamps, use of direct debits, etc.). For those with long-term mental illness or impairment, guardianship may need to be considered as an option to ensure adequate financial management.

Education

The proportion of school leavers without basic literacy/numeracy skills is increasing in the UK. Those from a non-English-speaking background will also be handicapped by inability to read leaflets, fill in forms, etc. Training in such basic skills, or learning English, can be the most important intervention a team makes. For those who have missed out on education through ill-health, flexible learning options, from part-time vocational courses to modular degrees, are now an option. Attending a class is also a valuable social opportunity.

Isolation

Isolation cannot be treated without an understanding of its cause. Social anxiety will need to be treated before a patient will be able to mix with others. Withdrawal due to depression is unlikely to improve without treatment of the depression. Those with poor English will need to be made aware of appropriate foreign language facilities. Isolation may need to be treated in a stepwise fashion, first by encouraging attendance at a team base or support group for those with similar illnesses, followed by supported attendance at community facilities, and eventually independent socialization.

Employment

Employment offers financial security, time structure, opportunities for social interaction and enhanced self-esteem. If a job has been stressful to the extent of being implicated in the aetiology of the patient's illness, stress management or relaxation techniques may be helpful in enabling the patient to cope better. For a patient with a long-term relapsing illness, careful attention may need to be paid to relapse signs so that suitable action can be taken before the patient's health deteriorates to a level that affects their work performance. Some employers are sympathetic to employees with mental illness and may be able to support a patient if their occupational health department has a knowledge of the patient's health and illness-management plan. It may be possible to find alternative employment in a less stressful job within the same company. For those who cannot remain in their current employment, or for the unemployed, government-sponsored job clubs may be helpful in advising a patient on suitable work opportunities.

Voluntary work can be a useful interim measure or an important step on the road to job readiness. For the more disabled, employment opportunities may be forthcoming through agencies such as the disablement resettlement officer, employment rehabilitation centres, skills training centres or initiatives set up by local mental health charities. Local branches of MIND often run cafés and shops staffed by those recovering from mental illness. In some areas, collectives are established by community mental health teams to run print shops, catering facilities and cleaning firms, which often network with local hospitals to gain contracts. If a member of the collective becomes unwell, another member will undertake to fulfil their duties. These collectives can be an important stepping stone for those aiming to return to full-time work.

Leisure

Again, the principle of accessing local community services is all-important. Many local authorities have leisure centres, gyms, swimming pools and activity centres that offer reduced rates to those claiming benefits. Non-vocational classes at local education centres can enable a patient to learn a new hobby or retrieve an old skill, and to meet other people simultaneously. A keyworker can also explore with the patient their desire for green spaces, via parks or day trips to the country, whether they would like to join a specific interest club, whether they would like penfriends, etc.

Transport

Those on low incomes, the mentally ill included, may be hampered in their pursuit of a full and active life by transport costs. Some local authorities are willing to give disabled-person travel passes to those suffering from mental illness. Railway and major bus companies often have special discount schemes or offers that can lessen the expense of travelling. For those who have become very isolated, it may be necessary for a team member to pick up patients from home in order to begin a process of rehabilitation in team base activities. Also, such activities should be planned for times when cheap travel is possible (out of commuter hours) and when nervous patients will not be put off by travelling after dark.

SOURCES OF SUPPORT

Self-help/support groups

Support groups are an important source of help for both patients and carers. They may be set up by a mental health team or may exist locally. If set up by professionals, they are an important opportunity for psychoeducation and for building a therapeutic alliance. Through a support group, patients can learn more about how others manage illness symptoms, and feel less isolated. Carers can network to maximize their knowledge of available resources, to socialize and to discover further coping strategies. Local MIND offices will have information about support groups, and the addresses for such organizations as the Manic Depressive Fellowship, the National Schizophrenia Association and others are listed at the end of this book.

Voluntary agencies

As well as nationally known charities, many areas have a network of voluntary agencies, and non-government organizations funded by social services, that can offer support and rehabilitation. Examples include schemes such as Crossroads, which offers practical help to carers, respite schemes, good neighbour schemes and organizations that provide holidays for those with long-term mental illness. Local libraries should have lists of all such agencies.

CONCLUSION

Social interventions should form part of any management plan in psychiatry. It is important to remember that both patients and their family or network of friends may need support. It is also important to achieve the right balance between positive encouragement and over-enthusiastic recommendations, which might overload a patient.

SECTION X

Useful Information

ADDRESSES

VOLUNTARY ORGANIZATIONS

Action on Phobias 8 The Avenue, Eastbourne, East Sussex BN21 3YA. Tel: 01321 53227

Afro-Caribbean Mental Health Association 35–37 Electric Avenue, London SW9 8JP. Tel: 020 7737 3603

Age Concern Astral House, 1268 London Road, London SW16 4ER Tel: 020 8765 7200 website: www.ageconcern.org.uk
Network of local organizations and over 100 national organizations in the UK and offer practical help information and advice

Agoraphobia Information Service 4 Manor Brook Road, London SE3 9AW Tel: 020 771 318 5026

Al-Anon/Alateen 61 Great Dover Street, London SE1 4YF. Helpline: 020 7403 0888 (24-hour), website: www.hexnet.co.uk/alanon
Support groups for the relatives and friends (Al-Anon) and children (Alateen) of problem drinkers

Alcohol Concern Waterbridge House, 32–36 Loman Street, London SE1 0EE. Tel: 020 7928 7377), website: www.alcoholconcern.org.uk
Alcohol counselling services

Alcoholics Anonymous PO Box 1, Stonebow House, Stonebow, York YO1 2NJ. Tel: 020 7352 3001, website: www.alcoholics-anonymous.org.uk
Helpline and national support network for those with drink problems

Alzheimer's Disease Society Gordon House, 10 Greencoat Place, London SW1P 1PH. Tel: 020 7306 0606, website: www.alzheimers.org.uk

Asian Family Counselling Service Rooms 4/5, 40 Equity Chambers, Piccadilly, Bradford; and 74 The Avenue, Ealing, London W13 8LB

Association for Post-Natal Illness 25 Jerdan Place, London SW6 1BE. Tel: 020 7386-0868, website: www.apni.org
Telephone helpline, information leaflets for sufferers and healthcare professionals as well as a network of volunteers who have themselves experienced postnatal illness

CancerBACUP (British Association of Cancer United Patients) 3 Bath Place, Rivington Street, London EC2A 3JR. Tel: 020 7608 1661, website: www.cancerbacup.org.uk

Carers National Association 20–25 Glasshouse Yard, London EC1A 4JT. Tel: 020 7490 8818, website: www.carersuk.demon.co.uk

Cot Death Society 7 Friars Walk, Thornby, Merseyside L37 4EU. Tel: 01704 870005

CRUSE – Bereavement Care Cruse House, 126 Sheen Road, Richmond, Surrey TW9 1UR. Tel: 0181 940 4818

Depression Alliance PO Box 1022, London SE1 7QB. Tel: 020 7721 7672, website: www.depressionalliance.org.uk
Help for people with depression, from organization run by sufferers themselves. Website contains information about the symptoms and treatments for depression, as well as Depression Alliance campaigns and local groups

Depressives Anonymous 36 Chestnut Avenue, Beverley, North Humberside, HU17 9QU. Tel: 01482 860619

Eating Disorders Association First Floor, Wensum House, 103 Prince of Wales Road, Norwich NR1 1DW. Helpline: 01603 621414 (9:00 to 18:30 weekdays), Youthline 01603 765050 (16:00 to 18:00 weekdays), website: www.edauk.com
Information and help on all aspects of eating disorders. Telephone helpline for people with an eating disorder, their family, friends, and professionals, along with a Youthline that offers information, help and support for young people aged 18 years and under. Network of support groups, postal and telephone contacts who offer support to those affected by eating disorders, throughout the UK

Families Anonymous Tel: 020 7498 4680, website: www.famanon.org.uk
For relatives and friends concerned about the use of drugs or related behavioural problems

Jewish Association for the Mentally Ill (JAMI) 16a North End Road, London NW11 7PH. Tel: 020 8458 2223, website: www.mentalhealth-jami.org.uk
Day care, social work, counselling advice, information and social activities for people suffering from severe mental illness

Making Space 46 Allen Street, Warrington WA2 7JB. Tel: 01925 571680
Self-help and carer support in the north of England

Manic Depression Fellowship Castle Works, 21 St George's Road, London SE1 6ES. Tel: 020 7793 2600, website: www.mdf.org.uk
Helps people affected by manic depression to take control of their lives. Information on bipolar disorder and support groups

Mental After-Care Association 25 Bedford Square, London WC1B 3HW. Tel: 020 7436 6194

MIND 15–19 Broadway, London E15 4BQ. Tel: 020 8519 2122, website: www.mind.org.uk
Leading mental health charity, working for a better life for everyone with experience of mental distress

Nafsiyat Intercultural Therapy Centre 278 Seven Sisters Road, Finsbury Park, London N4 2HY. Tel: 020 7263 4130

Narcotics Anonymous 202 City Road, London EC1V 2PH. Helpline: 020 7730 0009
Voluntary group for people with drug problems

National Association of Bereavement Services 20 Norton Felgate, Shoreditch, London E1 6DB. Tel: 020 7247 1080

National Association of Young Peoples' Counselling and Advice Services 11 Newarke Street, Leicester LE1 5SS. Tel: 01553 558763

National Autistic Society 393 City Road, London EC1V 1NG. Tel: 020 7833 2299, website: www.oneworld.org/autism_uk
Organization for people with autism and those who care for them, spearheading national and international initiatives

National Black Mental Health Association Macro House, 182 Soho Hill, Handsworth, Birmingham B19 1AF.

National Council of Voluntary Organisations Regent's Wharf, 8 All Saints Street, London N7 9RL. Tel: 020 7713 6161

National Phobics Society Zion Centre 339 Stretford Road, Hulme, Manchester M15 4ZY. Helpline: 0870 7700 456 (10:30am–4:00pm), website: www.phobics-society.org.uk/
User-led organization, run by sufferers and ex-sufferers of anxiety disorders

National Schizophrenia Fellowship 30 Tabernacle Street, London EC2A 4DD. Tel: 020 7330 9100, website: www.nsf.org.uk

NEWPIN St Margaret House, 21 Old Fort Road, London E2 9PL. Tel: 0181 980 3639

Refugee Support Centre King George House, Stockwell Road, London SW9 9ES. Tel: 0171 733 1482

RELATE Herbert Grey College, Little Church St, Rugby CV21 3AP. Tel: 01788 573241, website: www.relate.org.uk
Counselling, sex therapy, relationship education and training to support couple and family relationships throughout life

Re-Solv, Society for the Prevention of Solvent and Volatile Substance Abuse 30a High Street, Stone, Staffs ST15 8AW. Tel: 01785 817885

Richmond Fellowship for Community Mental Health 80 Holloway Road, London, N7 8JG. Tel: 020 7697 3300, website: www.richmondfellowship.org.uk
Care and rehabilitation for people with mental health needs in England and Wales

SAD Association PO Box 989, Steyning BN44 3HG. Tel: 01903 814 942, website: www.sada.org.uk
Support organization for seasonal affective disorder

Samaritans 17 Uxbridge Road, Slough SL1 1SN. Tel: 01753 532713, website: www.samaritans.org.uk
Confidential emotional support to any person who is suicidal or despairing

SANE (Schizophrenia A National Emergency) 2nd Floor, 199–205 Old Marylebone Road, London NW7 5QD. Tel: 020 7724 6520, SANELINE: 0845 767 8000, website: www.sane.org.uk
Telephone helpline (SANELINE) open 2pm–midnight every day of the year to give information and support on mental illness

Stillbirth and Perinatal Deaths Association Argyle House, 29–31 Euston Road, London NW1 2SD. 0171 833 2851

Survivors Speak Out 33 Lichfield Road, Cricklewood, London NW2

Terrence Higgins Trust BM AIDS, London WC1N 3XX. Tel: 020 7242 1010

Turning Point 101 Backchurch Lane, London E1 1LU.
Helpline: 020 7702 2300, website: www.turning-point.co.uk
Counselling for people with drug problems

United Kingdom Advocacy Network The Paddocks, Haggonsfields, Rhodesia, Worksop, Notts S80 3HW

VOICES 28 Castel Street, Kingston upon Thames, Surrey KT1 1SS.
Tel: 020 8547 3939
Groups for people who have experienced schizophrenia

OTHER USEFUL ADDRESSES

British Association for Counselling 1 Regent Place, Rugby CV21 2PJ.
Tel: 01788 578 328, website: www.counselling.co.uk
Promotes education and training for counsellors and the better understanding of counselling. Can provide lists of counselling services

British Association of Psychotherapists 37 Mapesbury Road, London NW2 4HJ. Tel: 020 8452 9823, website: www.bap-psychotherapy.org
Promotes education and training for psychotherapists. Also runs a clinical service with an initial consultation fee of £38. Subsequent fees negotiable. Minimum attendance three times a week for 2 years

British Psychological Society 48 Princess Road, Leicester LE1 7DR.
Tel: 01162 549 568, website: www.bps.org.uk
Gives information on and produces a directory of chartered psychologists throughout the UK

Mental Health Foundation 20/21 Cornwall Terrace, London NW1 4QL.
Tel: 020 7535 7400, website: www.mentalhealth.org.uk
Pioneering research and community projects aim to improve the support available for people with mental health problems and people with learning disabilities

PHENOMENOLOGY

In descriptive psychopathology, items are ordered as they would be encountered in writing down the mental state examination. Within each heading, items are listed alphabetically.

APPEARANCE AND BEHAVIOUR

General description of patient

What does the person look like? How are they dressed?

Abnormal postures

The general demeanour of the person is important: are they slumped in the chair sad and miserable, are they cowering fearfully in the corner or beaming expansively at the interviewer?

- **Perseveration of posture** is seen in schizophrenia, catalepsy and midbrain lesions
- **Waxy flexibility** is seen primarily in schizophrenia. When the person stops moving they maintain a fixed posture. It is also possible to place the person in a posture that they will maintain. Unlike catatonia the muscles are not contracted

Catatonia

Occurs in *catatonic schizophrenia* and is characterized by increased muscle tone. The person may exhibit no response to pain and may be incontinent.

Stupor

- **Akinetic mutism** is caused by space-occupying lesions of the third ventricle, thalamus and midbrain. The patient will appear alert with eyes open, exhibits a slight response to pain and has impaired registration and recall
- **Depressive stupor.** There is no catalepsy or incontinence and muscle tone is normal. Stupor may also be psychogenic

Movements

Goal-directed movements

- **Mannerisms** are abnormal, repetitive, goal-directed movements, such as a patient's arm describing a large arc every time a fork is used to pick up a mouthful of food
- **Obstruction** occurs when the person requires several attempts to complete an action. Sometimes they manage it, sometimes they don't. This is seen in catatonia and schizophrenia

Non-goal-directed movements

- **Athetoid movements** are slow, writhing, rotatory movements, particularly of the hands. The person may also assume unusual postures
- In **catatonic excitement,** the person shows senseless, apparently purposeless destructive behaviour while moving in a stilted fashion with deadpan features
- **Choreiform movements** are spontaneous, abrupt, random and jerky in nature and may resemble fragments of goal-directed actions. For example, someone with Huntington's chorea may be able to turn a jerky arm movement into scratching their head, or it may appear as if this was the intention. These movements can involve the trunk, limbs and face. Some actions also resemble snorting and sniffing. In Sydenham's chorea the movements are less jerky, tone is decreased and reflexes are prolonged
- **Gilles de la Tourette's syndrome** begins during childhood and involves tics of movement and verbal expression. There may be limb or facial tics such as grimacing or jumping, the sufferer will make repetitive grunting or barking noises and may exhibit *coprolalia* by shouting obscenities
- **Acute dystonias**, including **oculogyric crises**, can appear as tics or mannerisms
- **Parkinsonism**, including **pill-rolling tremor** and **cog-wheel rigidity**, may be iatrogenic
- **Spasmodic torticollis** involves involuntary contraction of the sternocleidomastoids
- **Stereotypies** are seen in normal people, schizophrenia, mental handicap and autism. The subject repeatedly performs the same movement, which may be simple, such as foot tapping, or more complex
- **Tardive dyskinesia** is usually due to antipsychotic medication. Look for orofacial dyskinesia, with lip smacking and tongue movements, and limb movements. Consider akathisia also as a cause of restlessness
- **Tics** may appear as expressive or defensive, usually facial, movements. They are seen in dystonia, after encephalitis and in Huntington's chorea and Gilles de la Tourette's syndrome
- **Tremor** characteristically involves the hands but may involve other parts of the body also. A resting tremor may be a normal 'essential' tremor resulting from anxiety, medication or alcohol. It may be the pill-rolling tremor of parkinsonism or the characteristic lip smacking and tremor of tardive dyskinesia. Intention tremor may point to cerebellar disease

Provoked movements

- **Automatic obedience** is a rare feature of schizophrenia, catatonia and dementia. The subject will literally obey any command automatically
- In **echopraxia**, the patient copies the interviewer's or other's movements. It is seen in schizophrenia, dementia, learning difficulty, epilepsy, anxiety in small children, transcortical aphasia and delirium
- **Forced grasping** is a symptom of frontal lobe disease. When shaking hands, the subject repeatedly takes and holds on to the proffered hand

- ***Mitgehen*** is seen in schizophrenia and organic brain conditions. When the subject is pushed, they move freely
- With ***mitmachen***, if the person is placed in a position they stay there
- **Negativism,** also called ***gegenhalten***, is seen in schizophrenia and organic brain disorders. It appears like passive resistance to movement and is not necessarily defensive or aggressive

MOOD

May be low (in depression) or elevated (in mania). The latter is often characterized by lability, or rapid mood swings. Lability is also seen in organic disorders, especially those affecting the frontal lobes. Irritability is a common feature of mood disturbance, especially mania.

- **Blunting** is a loss of the normal range of emotions, characterized by lack of reactivity. It is seen most frequently in chronic schizophrenia or when heavily medicated
- **Incongruency** is seen when mood or affect is at odds with what is being discussed or what is being described. In hebephrenic schizophrenia the affect is characteristically *fatuous*
- **Perplexity**, or anxious puzzled bewilderment, may characterize the prodromal or acute stages of schizophrenia
- **Alexithymia** (literally, no words to feel). Some people find it almost impossible to describe their emotions in words
- **Emotional indifference** is an extreme form of denial also known as *belle indifference*. Typically the person in hospital with a conversion disorder that leaves them paralysed will not seem at all bothered as staff try to establish the cause
- **Emotional incontinence** involves extreme lability of mood from moment to moment. It can be associated with organic conditions such as frontal lobe syndromes or pseudobulbar palsy

SPEECH AND THOUGHT

There may be specific difficulties in understanding or expressing thoughts, or in the articulation of speech.

- **Dysarthria** is disturbance of the articulation of speech because of muscle dysfunction
- **Dysphasia** is a disturbance of either the comprehension (receptive) or expression of speech, most commonly due to organic causes

It is helpful to think of the rate, volume and form of speech. The latter is often characterized by the manner in which thoughts are connected, the ability to maintain a single train of thought and the capacity to answer direct questions to the point. Specific psychiatric disorders have typical disorders of the form and content of speech associated with them. These constellations of signs and symptoms are indicative rather than pathognomonic.

- **Confabulation.** Asked what they had for breakfast that morning or for details of past psychiatric history, patients will tell a more or less plausible story that is completely invented. Due to severe impairment of short-term memory, as seen in Korsakoff's syndrome

The rate of speech is often disturbed in mood disorders. It may either be speeded up, in mania (**pressure of speech**), or slowed down, in depression (**psychomotor retardation**). True pressure of speech is very difficult to interrupt.

- **Flight of ideas** is characterized by a loss of coherent, goal-directed thinking with only obscure connections between ideas. Although often difficult to follow, and usually speeded up, it is possible to trace the train of ideas (unlike *loosening of associations*). Thoughts may be linked by rhyming, punning or alliteration (*clang associations*)

Schizophrenia

In acute schizophrenia there are a number of different approaches to discussing formal thought disorder. Bleuler described schizophrenia as a disorder of associations, of which loosening of associations is a manifestation. Schneider characterized schizophrenic thought disorder differently. He described five features (derailment, omission, substitution, fusion and drivelling), which come together to make three patterns: transitory, desultory and drivelling thinking. In addition, there are other terms used to describe other aspects of schizophrenic thought disorder.

Bleuler

- **Loosening of associations.** Bleuler used this term to describe condensation, displacement and the concrete use of symbols in schizophrenia
- **Condensation** is the incomprehensible combination of two or more ideas. It is difficult to distinguish from derailment and 'knight's move' thinking

Schneider

- **Derailment**: disrupted continuity and insertion of inappropriate material
- **Drivelling**: muddling of elements within an idea
- **Fusion**: merging and intertwining of ideas
- **Omission** of part or a whole thought
- **Substitution**: the main stream of thought is replaced by a secondary one

These five elements come together as:

- **Transitory thinking** – grammar and syntax are both affected
- **Desultory thinking** – grammar and syntax are correct but sudden ideas force their way into the stream of talk
- **Drivelling thinking** – parts of ideas become muddled up and the subject tries to unpick this

Other aspects

- **Concrete thinking.** A loss of the capacity for abstract thought; everything is taken very literally. One patient asked another 'Where are you from?' The other considered this for a moment and then replied 'I suppose I'm from my mother's tummy' and pointed at his abdomen to illustrate the point
- **Knight's move.** See *derailment* and *loosening of associations*
- **Neologisms**. The invention of new words or the attribution of new meanings to existing words. A patient described how people 'put the shine' on him. This neologistic use of 'shine' described how people read his thoughts and controlled his actions
- **Poverty of thought.** Often encountered with blunted affect and concrete thinking when negative symptoms are prominent
- **Thought block.** The sensation of the mind going blank is normal under stress, e.g. examinations. In thought block the sensation is of the train of thought 'hitting a brick wall' or being suddenly arrested
- **Word salad.** Meaningless verbigeration, as the name describes

Other disorders of speech and thinking

- **Echolalia.** Heard speech is repeated, usually only a word or phrase
- **Logoclonia.** A single syllable is repeated over and over, usually the last syllable of the last word. Seen in Parkinson's disease
- **Mutism.** Occurs in children, dissociative (conversion) disorder, depression, schizophrenia and organic syndromes
- **Palilalia**. A perseverated word is repeated faster and often
- **Perseveration.** A single word is repeated over and over again. It is not a stereotypy because the word was relevant to its context but persisted
- **Verbigeration** is a form of verbal stereotypy. Sentences, phrases or jargon are repeated for hours on end
- **Vorbeireden.** 'Talking past the point' is seen in Ganser's syndrome and acute schizophrenia

ABNORMAL PERCEPTIONS

Abnormal beliefs

Obsessions are impulses and thoughts that appear against the subject's will. They are recognized as a product of the subject's own mind, and resisting them initially increases anxiety. Resistance decreases with time. They may take the form of words, thoughts or images; their content may be sexual, religious, depressive, aggressive or concerning contamination or illness. They involve a single thought or image repeated over and over again.

Rumination involves worrying around a subject.

Primary delusions (synonyms: *autochthonous delusions* and *delusional perception*) come out of the blue in a two-stage process: a real perception or memory is suddenly invested with a delusional meaning. It may be preceded by a delusional mood. For example, a man went into a cafe. The person at the next table ordered macaroni cheese. The man, who had been perplexed for some time, suddenly realized that there was a homosexual conspiracy run by freemasons in the café. Primary delusions are a first-rank symptom of schizophrenia.

Secondary delusions derive from previous experiences; their onset is usually more insidious. They may relate to auditory hallucinations. Over time they can become systematized into an integrated set of beliefs. They are fixed, firm, unshakeable beliefs held in the face of evidence to the contrary and out of keeping with the subject's experience and context.

Systematized delusions are elaborated into a consistent world view by the subject. **Unsystematized delusions** do not 'fit' or have the same permanence. Circumscribed delusional systems may be held in such a way that the subject's lifestyle is not interfered with at all.

Delusions may also be characterized by their content – persecutory, grandiose, delusion of reference, erotic, religious, depressive, nihilistic, bizarre.

Overvalued ideas are intense preoccupations in which the subject has an emotional investment. They are not unshakeable and are usually false but understandable.

Disorders of self-awareness

- **Anosognosia.** Denial or lack of awareness of paralysis or sensory deficit
- **Depersonalization** describes the sensation that one is not real or not really there. It occurs in anxiety states, schizophrenia, epilepsy, depression and organic disorders
- **Derealization** involves the sense that one's surroundings are dull, flat and somehow not real
- **Distorted body image**: in anorexia, sufferers believe themselves to be overweight – typically with 'enormous thighs' – when they are actually emaciated. Some debate whether or not this is a delusion

Passivity phenomena

These are disorders of the possession of thought and involve loss of the sense of boundaries between the self and the world.

- **Made actions**. The subject's physical actions are under external control: the sense is of being radio-controlled or having to respond in a particular way when a certain external event occurs
- **Thought broadcast.** This is an example of the loss of the boundaries of the self. The subject feels that their thoughts are available to other people. They may be broadcast over the radio or via television aerials
- **Thought insertion.** An outside agency puts alien thoughts into the subject's mind
- **Thought withdrawal.** Thoughts are removed as if by a vacuum cleaner. This can be differentiated from thought block by asking: 'Do you ever find that your thoughts stop dead and leave your mind a complete blank?' (thought block) and 'Do you ever find that people can interfere with your thoughts or read your mind?' (passivity)

Perceptual disturbances

Sensory distortions

- **Dysmegalopsia.** Distortion of spatial form occurring with retinal scarring and temporal lobe disorders
- **Hyperacusis.** Extreme sensitivity to sounds, as in mania and hyperthyroidism
- **Hypoacusis** occurs in delirium
- **Micropsia.** Things appear smaller than they are
- **Xanthopsia.** Changes in colour vision, usually drug-induced. May also occur in temporal lobe epilepsy and erythopsia from retinal haemorrhage

Sensory deceptions

Eidetic imagery is vivid visual recall of previous perception, usually occurring in the mind's eye: 'photographic memory'

Illusions are misperceptions of external events, such as seeing a tree in the dark and thinking it is a person. Seeing lines on wallpaper turn into snakes in delirium tremens is also an example of this

Pareidolia is a type of illusion in which pictures are seen in the fire or in the clouds. It implies the creation of vivid mental images without effort

Pseudohallucinations. This term is used in two ways. Jaspers used it to describe vivid mental images, a form of eidetic imagery or variant of fantasy. The perception is located in the mind, not in external space and is not consciously manipulated. Hare used the term to describe perceptions in the absence of an external perception that nevertheless appear to be located in the real world – but which the subject recognizes as not real

Hallucinations are perceptions occurring in the absence of an external stimulus. They are perceived as if occurring in the real world and thus have the same qualities as real perceptions. They occur in schizophrenia, mood disorders, dissociative states, delirium, dementia and other brain disorders, and in normal people. They may be formed or unformed and in any sensory modality. Obtaining a description of a hallucination is rather like getting a patient to describe a pain or a lump: what modality is it? Formed or unformed? If voices, one or several? Strangers or familiar voices? Where are they located? What are they saying? What is its effect?, etc.

- **Auditory.** May be elementary, with fragments of sounds, music or voices, or fully formed. In psychotic depression they are usually *second-person* and derogatory or urging the sufferer to harm themselves. In schizophrenia they are characteristically *third-person,* discussing the sufferer or providing a running commentary, although second-person voices also occur. Voices may provide a *running commentary* on the subject. *Thought echo* is a first-rank symptom of schizophrenia. It is a type of auditory hallucination in which the subject reports hearing their thoughts echoed inside their head or outside it
- **Autoscopy** is the ability to step outside one's body and see oneself. It can occur in extreme anxiety but is more commonly associated with intoxication with alcohol or drugs, delirium and epilepsy. In the myth of the *Doppelgänger* it is part of a near-death experience

- **Extracampine hallucinations** occur outside the sensory field. One is able to see and hear people in another town
- **Functional hallucination.** A stimulus in one modality causes a hallucination; both are experienced. A woman reported hearing God talking to her when the clock chimed. It occurs in schizophrenia
- **Pain and deep sensation.** Twisting and tearing sensations inside the body occur in chronic schizophrenia. *Delusional zoopathy* is the sensation that an animal is living inside one's body. It can occur in pellagra, thalamic tumours and schizophrenia
- **Reflex hallucination.** An event perceived in one sensory modality leads to a consequence in another. When sneezing, the patient experiences a pain in the leg
- **Taste and smell.** Hallucinations in these modalities are rare and occur in temporal lobe epilepsy, irritation of the olfactory bulb, schizophrenia and delirium
- **Touch.** *Formication* is the sensation of having insects crawling in or under the skin. It is also called delusional infestation and can be caused by cocaine or alcohol withdrawal. *The cocaine bug* consists of formication plus persecutory delusions
- **Vestibular hallucinations** produce the sensation of flying through the air or falling back through the bed. They occur in normal people but also in substance abuse and intoxication, psychosis and delirium
- **Visual hallucinations** may be elementary (flashes), partly organized (patterns) or fully organized. They are found in delirium, dissociative states, substance abuse and other brain disorders. Lilliputian hallucinations are pleasant visual hallucinations of little people or objects that occur in delirium. LSD produces sensory distortions such as synaesthesia, where one can, for example, hear colours, rather than hallucinations

INSIGHT

This has many components beyond attitude to treatment and diagnosis. It includes recognition of illness and awareness that mental illness is a plausible explanation for present experiences. The patient should also be asked about their views of the value of compliance and the implications of their illness and its effects on self and others.

PSYCHIATRIC RATING SCALES

Standardized instruments are commonly used in psychiatric research and practice for identifying psychiatric 'cases', improving the accuracy of assessment and diagnosis, assessing the severity of psychiatric symptoms and social disabilities, and evaluating change in response to specific interventions.

There are three main types of instrument: self-report, interview-based and observational assessments. The choice between these depends on the purpose for which it is intended, the condition under investigation, the setting in which the study will take place, the nature of the information to be gathered, the sample size, and the time and resources available for data collection. If an interview-based measure is to be used, a further choice must be made between an instrument suitable for use by lay interviewers and one that requires specialist clinical skills.

The psychometric properties of psychiatric instruments can be considered under the headings of reliability and validity. Since there are no 'gold standards' by which to assess the validity of psychiatric instruments, great store has been set by developing instruments that are reliable. It must be remembered that, while important, reliability is really of secondary significance: it is necessary but not sufficient for establishing the validity of an instrument.

Reliability refers to the repeatability of measurement. A reliable instrument is one that produces the same results on repeated administration. There are three formal criteria by which the reliability of instruments is traditionally assessed: *inter-rater* (the level of agreement between two raters), *test–retest* (agreement between scores for the same subject over time), and *split-half reliability* (a measure of the internal consistency of an instrument).

Validity is defined as the extent to which an instrument measures what it claims to measure. There are five main types of validity: *face validity* (the general appearance of the instrument), *content validity* (whether an instrument appears to be a balanced and comprehensive measure of the phenomenon of interest), *criterion validity* (a measure of agreement between an instrument and an external criterion), *construct validity* (the extent to which results obtained using an instrument are consistent with theoretical assumptions underlying its design) and *predictive validity* (the extent to which scores on an instrument are predictive of some future event).

INSTRUMENTS IN COMMON USE

Case-finding instruments

The aims of epidemiological investigation include estimating the frequency and distribution of disorder in populations and searching for potential aetiological risk factors. Any such enquiry requires a definition of 'caseness' and instruments capable of accurately identifying 'cases'. It must be remembered, however, that most populations contain subjects with symptoms ranging from the transient and minor to the severe and chronic, and any definition of 'caseness' amounts to the imposition of a threshold value on a continuous distribution. The current definition of a 'case' of psychiatric disorder is that the patient's symptoms fulfil the operational criteria of DSM-IV or ICD-10.

The most widely used case-finding instrument in the UK is the ***General Health Questionnaire (GHQ)***.[1] The GHQ was developed on the assumption that there are undifferentiated subjective experiences of psychiatric disorder that distinguish all such patients from those who are well. The questionnaire was originally intended for use in primary-care settings and enquires about recent changes in functioning. The resulting score is a quantitative assessment of the likelihood that an individual would be identified as a psychiatric case by a psychiatrist. The GHQ is highly acceptable to the general population and has been extensively validated.

An alternative is the ***Self-Reporting Questionnaire (SRQ)***,[2] a 24-item questionnaire developed by the World Health Organization for use in developing countries. The SRQ is as effective in case detection as the GHQ, and Yes/No response categories make it particularly suitable in settings where literacy may be poor.

Assessment of global psychopathology

The ***Present State Examination (PSE)*** was first published in 1967[3] and has now reached its 10th edition. A computer program, CATEGO, was developed in 1971 to produce standardized diagnostic groupings. The PSE is designed for use by psychiatrists after a specified period of training. Interviewers are trained to discover whether each of a comprehensive list of symptoms is present, and if so with what degree of severity. For most symptoms questions are suggested, but interviewers are free to clarify with their own supplementary questions when necessary. For the ninth edition of the PSE an index of definition (ID) was constructed based on the number, type and severity of symptoms elicited. The index specifies eight levels of definition of disorder, and the threshold for 'caseness' is set between levels 4 and 5.

PSE 10 has been incorporated into the ***Schedule for Clinical Assessment in Neuropsychiatry (SCAN)***.[4] SCAN represents a comprehensive procedure for clinical examination capable of generating ICD-10, DSM-III-R and DSM-IV categories. A major addition to PSE 10 is the inclusion of sections on eating disorders, somatoform disorders and alcohol and substance abuse, which were absent from PSE 9. SCAN contains a 59-item group checklist, consisting of groups of symptoms, and a clinical information schedule for use with case records, carers and other informants. SCAN also gives the option of supplementing information on present state by rating a secondary period, which can be a previous representative episode of illness or a lifetime rating.

The ***Composite International Diagnostic Interview (CIDI)*** is a standardized instrument designed for use by lay interviewers in epidemiological studies in crosscultural settings.[5] The CIDI combines items from the PSE and the ***Diagnostic Interview Schedule (DIS),***[6] an instrument used by lay interviewers in the Epidemiological Catchment Area study. Data gathered using the CIDI are sufficient to make reliable ICD-10 and DSM-IV diagnoses. Both the DIS and CIDI ask first about lifetime prevalence of symptoms, before enquiring about timing of onset and duration to arrive at lifetime, 1-year, 6-month and 3-month prevalence rates. The main advantages of CIDI are its standardization, extensive field testing in diverse settings and languages, and exceptionally high reliability. The main drawbacks of the CIDI are the time needed for training and the duration of the interview, which lasts for over 2 hours in one-third of cases. There are now several versions of the CIDI, including 12-month, short-form (CIDI-SF), primary health care (CIDI-PHC) and computer-administered (CIDI-Auto).

The ***Clinical Interview Schedule (CIS)***[7] was the first standardized interview designed to assess common mental disorders in community settings among subjects who may not see themselves as psychiatrically disturbed. In its original form, the CIS resembled a clinical interview and required the interviewer to judge whether the subject was a psychiatric case and to decide on an appropriate diagnosis. High reliability was obtained among trained raters. The CIS has been revised (***CIS-R***) for use by lay interviewers,[8] by removing all but the standardized enquiry into non-psychotic symptoms. Elimination of the 'manifest abnormality' section means that it is largely free from observer bias and is less dependent on training. While extending its applicability in non-psychiatric settings, these changes did not alter the validity of the CIS. A computerized version of this instrument has been shown to possess psychometric properties similar to the original.

The ***Brief Psychiatric Rating Scale (BPRS)***[9] was designed to assess treatment efficacy in psychopharmacological research, and has been used most widely among patients with psychotic disorders. The BPRS consists of 18 symptom constructs rated on a seven-point scale of severity. Reliability is high among clinically experienced raters within centres, but lack of cues for rating severity leads to variation between centres. The most serious drawbacks are the overlap between items and their lack of correspondence with current psychopathological concepts, making ratings susceptible to the halo effect.

The ***Schedule for Affective Disorders and Schizophrenia (SADS)***[10] is a semi-structured interview for use by experienced clinicians and was the most widely used diagnostic instrument in psychiatric research in the USA prior to the advent of DSM-III. This interview was designed for use with psychiatric patients and provides a comprehensive assessment of the symptoms of disorders defined by the Research Diagnostic Criteria (RDC). The full SADS interview enquires separately about the time of maximum symptom severity during the current episode, the severity of symptoms in the past week, and lifetime experience of symptoms. Other versions of the SADS include the SADS-L (lifetime version) and the SADS-C (change version), which is suitable for repeated administration with the same subject.

The ***Structured Interview for DSM-IV (SCID)***[11] is a DSM-IV-compatible version of the SADS that requires less training than the original. Unlike the SADS, the SCID incorporates diagnostic algorithms within the interview. Questions are grouped by diagnosis and if any criterion essential to a diagnosis is not met the interviewer is instructed to skip the remaining questions about that diagnosis. Like the SADS, interviewers are encouraged to gather information from as many sources as possible. Versions of the SCID include SCID-II, which assesses personality disorders, SCID-P (patient), a self-report version for use among those identified as psychiatric patients, and SCID-NP (non-patient), for use where subjects are not necessarily seeking help for psychiatric disorders.

Assessment of the severity of specific conditions

Depression

More instruments have been developed for the assessment of depression than for any other psychiatric disorder; a recent review[12] identified over 30 in the English language alone. Of these, the most commonly used are listed below.

The ***Hamilton Rating Scale for Depression (HRSD)***,[13] an observer scale consisting of 17 (or, less commonly, 21) items scored on a combination of five- and three-point scales. Designed for use by experienced clinicians, training in the use of this instrument is necessary. There are no standardized questions but a detailed glossary is provided. The instrument assesses cognitive and behavioural aspects of depression but places particular emphasis on somatic symptoms.

The ***Beck Depression Inventory (BDI)***[14] is a 21-item self-report measure that assesses sadness, anhedonia, suicidal ideation, negative cognitions and somatic manifestations of depression. Like the HRSD, the BDI should only be used to assess severity once a diagnosis of depression has been made. No training in its use is necessary and it is suitable for frequent use on the same subject.

The ***Montgomery–Asberg Depression Rating Scale (MADRS)***[15] was designed to assess change in severity of depression. The MADRS consists of 10 items, none of which concerns somatic or psychomotor symptoms.

The ***Hospital Anxiety and Depression Scale (HAD)***[16] was originally intended for use in general medical settings, where scores on other instruments may be contaminated by symptoms of physical illness. The HAD comprises two seven-item self-report scales. Items on the depression scale are largely restricted to the assessment of anhedonia, although anxiety items enquire about autonomic symptoms. The HAD should be used with care in applications other than that for which it was designed.

Eating disorders

The ***Eating Attitudes Test (EAT)***[17] is a self-report instrument consisting of 26 items covering both cognition and behaviour. EAT score is dominated by a 'dieting' component, making it difficult to interpret except among those who are thin or pathologically preoccupied with their weight.[18] Although validated as a measure of the severity of anorexia nervosa, the EAT has also been used inappropriately for case identification in community surveys. Used in this way, the EAT has a positive predictive value of around 10%, since the prevalence of this disorder is less than 1%. The EAT is further limited by the tendency of anorexic subjects to deny their illness.

Personality disorder

The ***Eysenck Personality Inventory (EPI)***[19] is the personality questionnaire most widely used in the UK. Its 48 questions measure two major orthogonal factors: extraversion/introversion (E) and neuroticism (N). The test also incorporates a lie scale. Twin studies demonstrate that both E and N are moderately heritable.

Standardized interviews based on the operational definitions of personality disorder found in ICD-10 and DSM-IV such as the ***Personality Assessment Schedule (PAS)***[20] and the ***Standardised Assessment of Personality (SAP)***[21] have allowed systematic research into the prevalence rate of personality disorders, their impact upon outcome for other clinical disorders and the validity of the various subcategories of personality disorder.

INSTRUMENTS USED IN SOCIAL PSYCHIATRY

Assessment of social functioning

Social disabilities associated with psychiatric disorder can be more distressing for a patient than specific symptoms. Social impairments may be longer lasting and harder to treat, and social functioning may be a better predictor of service utilization and cost of care than either diagnosis or symptomatology.

The ***Global Assessment of Functioning Scale (GAF)*** was introduced as axis V of DSM-III-R, to provide a measure of 'a person's psychological, social and occupational functioning'.[22] The GAF is a modified version of the ***Global Assessment Scale (GAS)***,[23] which has been widely used in both research and clinical settings and has established reliability. Using nine anchor points describing different levels of symptoms and functioning, the rater decides on a single number between 0 and 90 to summarize a person's overall condition. Although simple, combining symptoms and functioning in a single rating may be misleading or uninformative.

A more precise measure of current functioning is obtained by examining a person's recent performance in specific social roles. The ***MRC Social Role Performance Schedule (SRP)***[24] compares individual functioning with population norms, although it must be remembered that some roles may be inappropriate for certain study populations. For instance, prisoners or institutionalized patients will not have the opportunity to fulfil domestic, sexual or financial roles. The ***Social Behaviour Scale (SBS)***[25] measures a range of behaviours, mainly on five-point scales, and has established psychometric properties.

OTHER MEASURES RELEVANT TO PSYCHIATRY

Quality of life

Quality of life is notoriously difficult to define. The major components are the absence of symptoms, adequate social performance and the ability to engage in satisfying activities. Two examples of quality of life measures suitable for people with mental disorders are the ***Quality of Life Interview***[26] and the ***Lancashire Quality of Life Schedule***.[27]

Needs assessment

People with serious mental illness frequently have a complex mix of medical and social needs. In the UK, recent government policy has placed great emphasis on the assessment of individual need prior to the planning and delivery of care. Regular clinical assessments of patients' needs are essential for the appropriate targeting of care. Measurement of met and unmet need is a powerful outcome measure for any mental health service evaluation. The ***MRC Needs for Care Assessment (NCA)*** identifies potentially remediable areas in which a patient's level of functioning is at or below a minimum specified level.[24] The ***Camberwell Assessment of Need (CAN)***[28] is a more recently developed instrument, which is briefer than the NCA and is suitable for use by untrained raters. This instrument covers 22 social and clinical needs. Levels of met and unmet need are recorded, along with measures of the amount of help received from informal carers and health professionals. Each item is rated independently by the subject and their keyworker.

REFERENCES

1. Goldberg DP. Detecting psychiatric illness by questionnaire. Maudsley Monograph 22. Oxford: Oxford University Press, 1972.
2. Harding TW, de Arango MV, Baltazar J et al. Mental disorders in primary health care: a study of their frequency and diagnosis in four developing countries. Psychol Med 1980; 10: 231–241.
3. Wing JK, Birley JLT, Cooper JE et al. Reliability of a procedure for measuring and classifying 'present psychiatric state'. Br J Psychiatry 1967; 113: 499–515.
4. Wing JK, BaborT, Brugha T et al. SCAN. Arch Gen Psychiatry 1990; 47: 589–593.
5. Robins LN, Sartorius N. Editorial. Int J Methods Psychiatr Res 1993; 3: 63–65.
6. Robins LN, Helzer JE, Croughan J et al. National Institute of Mental Health Diagnostic Interview Schedule: its history, characteristics and validity. Arch Gen Psychiatry 1981; 38: 381–389.
7. Goldberg DP, Cooper B, Eastwood MR et al. A standardised psychiatric interview for use in community settings. Br J Prevent Soc Med 1970; 24: 18–23.
8. Lewis G, Pelosi AJ, Araya R et al. Measuring psychiatric disorder in the community: a standardised assessment for use by lay interviewers. Psychol Med 1992; 22, 465–486.
9. Overall JE, Gorham DR. The Brief Psychiatric Rating Scale (BPRS). Psychol Rep 1962; 10: 799–812.
10. Endicott J, Spitzer RL. A diagnostic interview: the Schedule for Affective Disorders and Schizophrenia. Arch Gen Psychiatry 1978; 3: 837–844.
11. Spitzer RL, Williams JBW, Gibbon M et al. The Structured Clinical Interview for DSM-III-R (SCID). I: History, rationale and description. Arch Gen Psychiatry 1992; 49: 624–629.
12. Snaith P. What do depression rating scales measure? Br J Psychiatry 1993; 163: 293–298.
13. Hamilton M. A rating scale for depression. J Neurol Neurosurg Psychiatry 1960; 23: 56–62.
14. Beck AT, Ward CH, Mendelson M et al. An inventory for measuring depression. Arch Gen Psychiatry 1961; 4: 561–571.
15. Montgomery SA, Asberg M. A new depression scale designed to be sensitive to change. Br J Psychiatry 1979; 134: 382–389.
16. Zigmond AS, Snaith RP. The Hospital Anxiety and Depression Scale. Acta Psychiatr Scand 1982; 67: 361–370.
17. Garner DM, Garfinkel PE. The Eating Attitudes Test: an index of the symptoms of anorexia nervosa. Psychol Med 1979; 9: 273–279.

18. Wells JE, Cooper PA, Gabb DC, Pears PK. The factor structure of the eating attitudes test with adolescent schoolgirls. Psychol Med 1985; 15: 141–146.
19. Eysenck HJ, Eysenck SBG. Manual of Eysenck Personality Inventory. London: University of London Press, 1964.
20. Tyrer P, Alexander J. Classification of personality disorder. Br J Psychiatry 1979; 135: 163–167.
21. Mann AH, Jenkins R, Cutting JC. The development and use of a standardised assessment of abnormal personality. Psychol Med 1981; 11: 839–847.
22. American Psychiatric Association. DSM-III-R. Washington, DC: American Psychiatric Association, 1987. In UK available from The Press Syndicate, University of Cambridge, Trumpington St, Cambridge CB2 1RP.
23. Endicott J, Spitzer RL, Fleiss JL et al. The global assessment scale. Arch Gen Psychiatry 1976; 33: 766–771.
24. Brewin C, Wing J, Mangen S et al. Principles and practice of measuring needs in the long-term mentally ill: the MRC Needs of Care Assessment. Psychol Med 1987; 17: 971–982.
25. Wykes T, Sturt E. The measurement of social behaviour in psychiatric patients: an assessment of the reliability and validity of the SBS schedule. Br J Psychiatry 1986; 148: 1–11.
26. Lehman A. The well-being of chronic mental patients – assessing their quality of life. Arch Gen Psychiatry 1982; 40: 369–374.
27. Oliver JPJ. The Social Care Directive: development of a quality of life profile for use in community services for the mentally ill. Soc Work Soc Sci Rev 1991; 3: 5–45.
28. Thornicroft G, Ward P, James S. Care management and mental health. Br Med J 1993; 20: 768–771.

INDEX